DESTINY'S STYLE

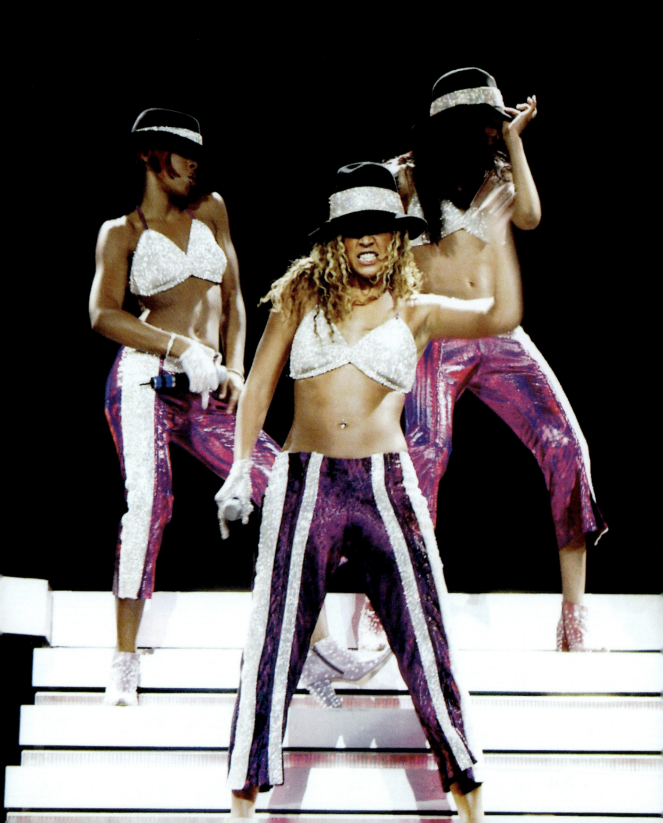

DESTINY'S STYLE

BOOTYLICIOUS FASHION, BEAUTY, AND LIFESTYLE SECRETS FROM DESTINY'S CHILD

tina knowles with zoë alexander

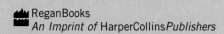

ReganBooks
An Imprint of HarperCollinsPublishers

DESTINY'S STYLE. Copyright © 2002 by Tina Knowles. All rights reserved. Printed in the United States of America. No part of this book may be used or reproduced in any manner whatsoever without written permission except in the case of brief quotations embodied in critical articles and reviews. For information address HarperCollins Publishers Inc., 10 East 53rd Street, New York, NY 10022.

HarperCollins books may be purchased for educational, business, or sales promotional use. For information please write: Special Markets Department, HarperCollins Publishers Inc., 10 East 53rd Street, New York, NY 10022.

FIRST EDITION

Designed by Platinum Design, Inc. NYC

Printed on acid-free paper

Library of Congress Cataloging-in-Publication Data
Knowles, Tina.
    Destiny's style: bootylicious fashion, beauty, and lifestyle secrets from Destiny's Child / Tina Knowles, with Zöe Alexander.
      p. cm
  ISBN 0-06-009777-9
    1. Destiny's Child (Musical group) 2. Rock musicians—Costume—History. 3. Costume design. 4. Rock music—History and criticism. I. Alexander, Zöe. II. Title.
ML421.D47.K66 2002
782.421643'092'2—dc21   2002021267

02 03 04 05 06   WBC/RRD   10 9 8 7 6 5 4 3 2 1

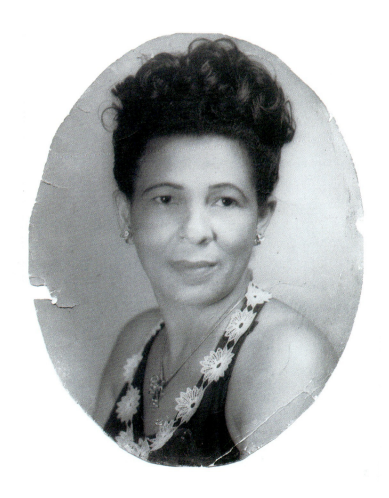

This book is dedicated to my mother, Agnes Dereon Beyoncé, where it all started. And to Johnny Rittenhouse—the world is a much less funny and creative place without you. I love you both. Rest in peace.

CONTENTS

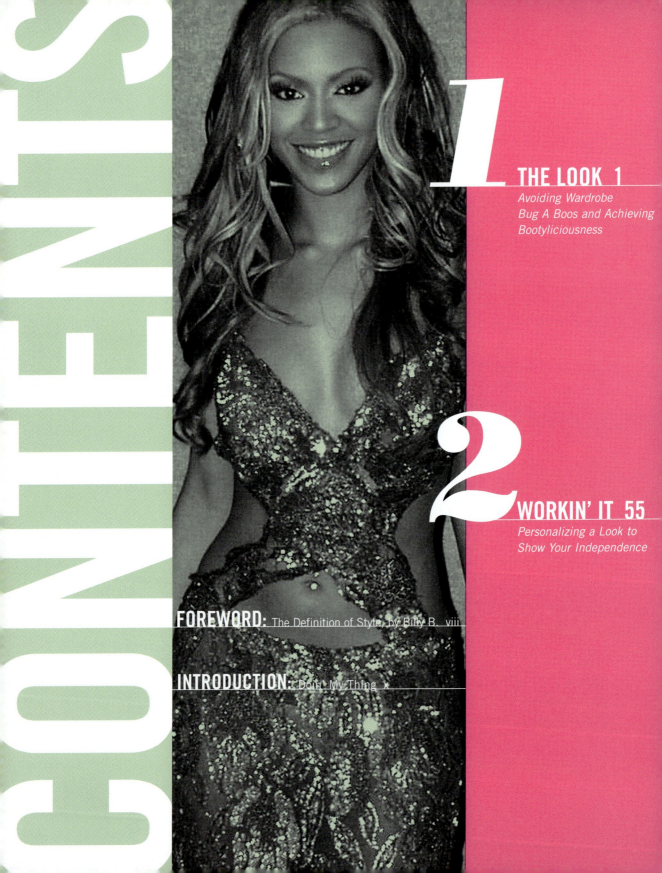

1 THE LOOK 1
Avoiding Wardrobe Bug A Boos and Achieving Bootyliciousness

2 WORKIN' IT 55
Personalizing a Look to Show Your Independence

FOREWORD: The Definition of Style, by Billy B. viii

INTRODUCTION: Doin' My Thing x

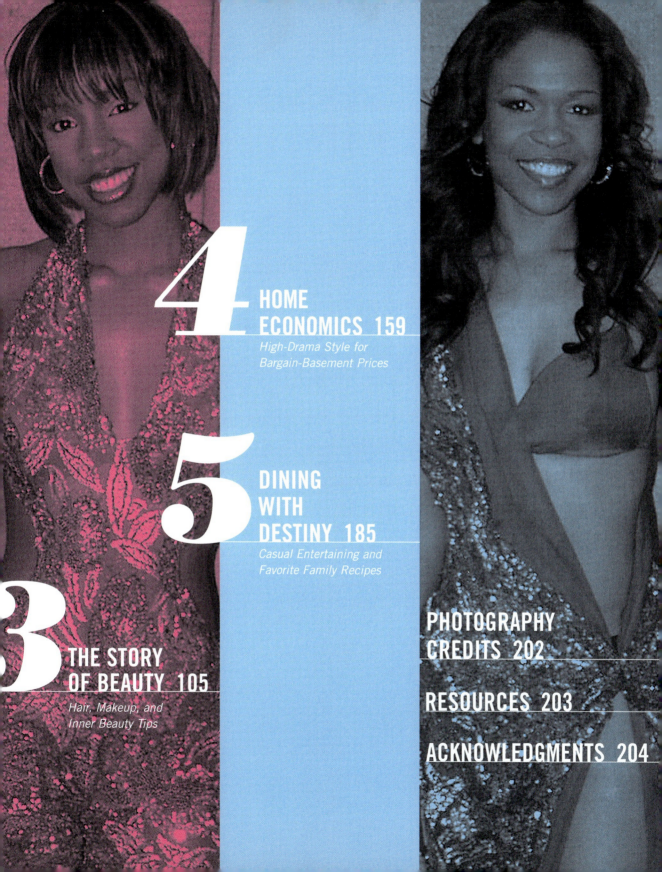

4 HOME ECONOMICS 159
High-Drama Style for Bargain-Basement Prices

5 DINING WITH DESTINY 185
Casual Entertaining and Favorite Family Recipes

3 THE STORY OF BEAUTY 105
Hair, Makeup, and Inner Beauty Tips

PHOTOGRAPHY CREDITS 202

RESOURCES 203

ACKNOWLEDGMENTS 204

FOREWORD

THE DEFINITION OF STYLE

Oxford Dictionary:

Style: A way of doing something. A distinctive appearance, design, or arrangement.

Stylist: A person who designs clothes or cuts hair.

Random House–Webster's Handy American Dictionary:

Stylist: A person who cultivates a distinctive style.

Webster's New Dictionary of the English Language:

Style: Elegant or fashionable way of living.

THESE DEFINITIONS DESCRIBE TINA TO A *T*! THEY SHOULD INCLUDE AS PART OF THEIR DEFINITION OF STYLE "SEE TINA KNOWLES" (MAYBE ONE DAY THEY WILL).

It's hard to describe what a good stylist is. I think anybody can go see a fashion show, take an outfit directly from the runway, and put it on someone else. That's not being a stylist, that's dressing someone. Good stylists take a piece from here and a piece from there and put it together to create a style that's all their own and suits their clients. Or better yet, a stylist starts from scratch and builds a look from the floor up. That's precisely what Tina does! And when I say "from scratch," I mean from scratch!

Tina's the kind of stylist who, in a pinch (and during the four years I've worked with her, I've seen her in many), can take a fifteen-dollar pair of shoes and with a little time, a glue gun, and a Bedazzler can turn those suckers into a pair of shoes that would rival Manolo

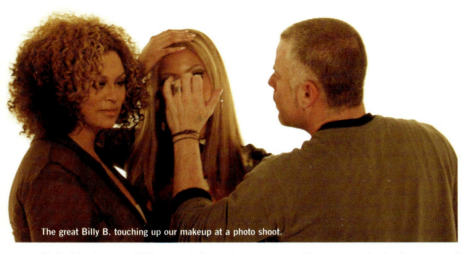

The great Billy B. touching up our makeup at a photo shoot.

> "she is dedicated and selfless"

Blahnik's. I mean, if Tina needed to, she would rip the drapes right off the window and whip up a fabulous gown in no time! No problem. She is truly a modern-day Scarlett O'Hara.

Before writing this, I called Beyoncé, Kelly, and Michelle to ask them to help me recall the most extreme example of Tina making something out of nothing because their luggage was lost, or the clothes didn't fit properly, or FedEx didn't arrive on time. We laughed because there have been so many times, we couldn't pick just one. Actually, it's abnormal when there *isn't* a style emergency. It's the nature of the beast.

There was one time—soon after Tina, Mathew, and their family had moved into their new home and didn't have a stick of furniture in it—that MTV Cribs was scheduled to film Destiny's Child at home. Two weeks before MTV came, the girls had to travel to Japan, but Tina returned to Houston and completely decorated the entire home—complete with a custom Moroccan-style bedroom—and MTV filmed as scheduled. As if that wasn't enough, immediately following that, I was part of a crew (I did the makeup) that came to their home to shoot a magazine cover. Not only did Tina have the house ready for the photo shoot but she also designed the clothes, did the hair, and prepared the meanest pot of gumbo to rival Emeril Lagasse.

But of all the examples, I decided this was the one that really sums it all up: Tina was doing the girls' hair for an event and thought highlights would look great with their outfits. The only problem was that there wasn't enough time to start highlighting, so she clipped pieces of her own beautiful honey-colored locks and carefully pinned them into their hair, one section at a time. The girls fought her all the way, telling her *"Don't cut your hair!"* Tina replied, "Oh, it's just hair, it'll grow back." She is that dedicated and selfless, not only as a stylist but also as a wife, mother, and friend.

—**Billy B.,**
celebrity makeup artist

INTRODUCTION

DOIN' MY THING

WHEN I WAS FIRST APPROACHED TO DO A BOOK ABOUT STYLE, I HAD SERIOUS RESERVATIONS.

I thought, "Who am I to write a book on style?" It's true that I've been designing and making clothes since I was a teenager, and that my clothes have appeared in Destiny's Child videos, in international fashion magazines, and on the red carpet at numerous celebrity events. I've decorated homes and offices that have been featured in the media. But a *book?* What a daunting task for someone like me, who already juggles so many things. From owning a hair salon, working as the wardrobe stylist for both Destiny's Child and my youngest daughter, Solange, and designing clothes for my clothing company to being a wife and mother, my plate is more than full. My inner critic filled me with doubt about being able to pull off a book like this because, aside from having very little free time, I wasn't formally trained in fashion and style. Unlike most professional designers and wardrobe stylists I have never set foot in a fashion or design school. I'm an oddity in my business, which used to bother me because there are some people who never let you forget that you're not "classically" trained from some hoity-toity fashion or design school. For a long time it made me a little insecure. But then I realized that everything about my life and the career paths I've chosen has been very risky, unique, and eclectic—which is how some have described my style. Finally, my wonderful husband, Mathew, who saw me struggling with the decision to write a book, looked at me and said, "Tina, you can do this." Now, most people who know my husband, personally or even just by reputation, know that when he thinks something is a good idea—it usually is. So I took a deep breath and decided to get on out there and "do my thing."

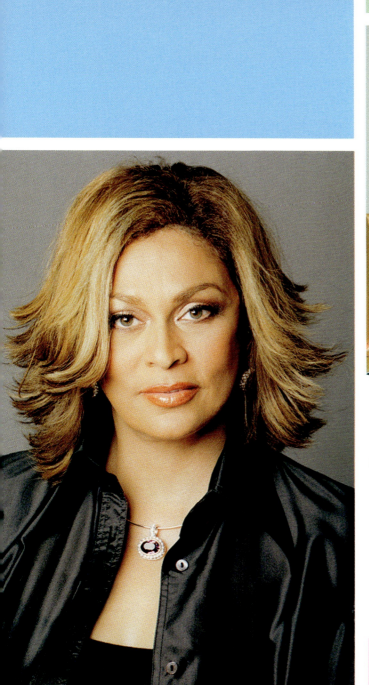

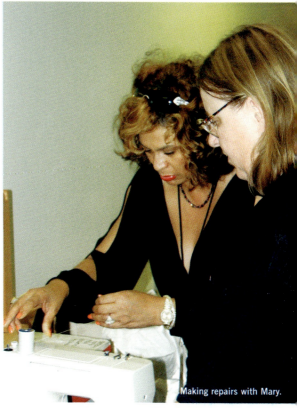

Making repairs with Mary.

" it's true that i've been designing and making clothes since i was a teenager"

INTRODUCTION | xi

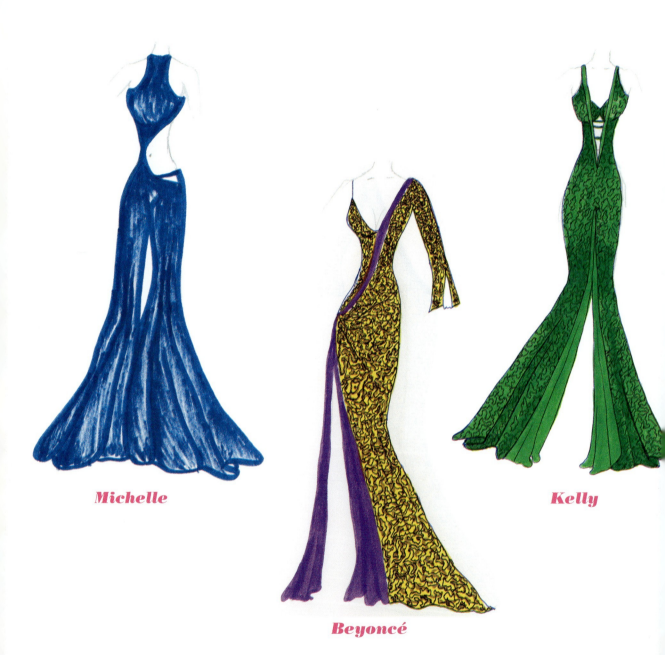

My sketches for what each girl would wear to the fifteenth Soul Train Music Awards. I kept their personalities in mind when designing each one.

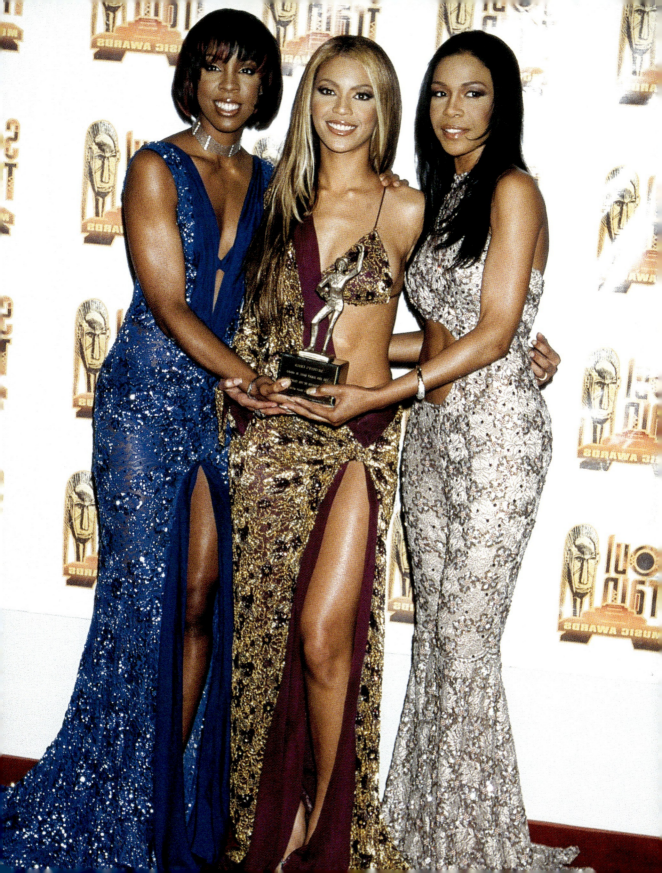

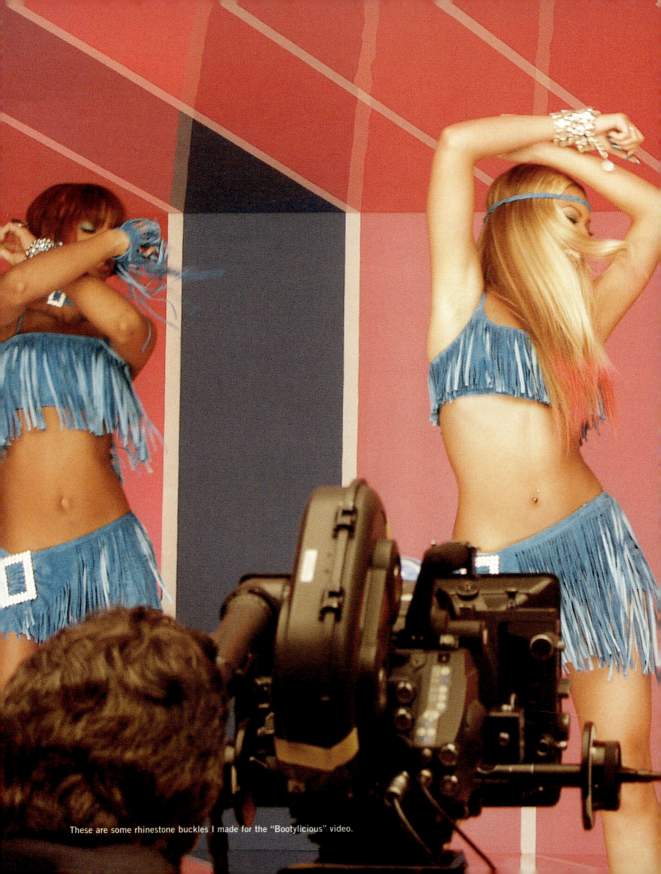

These are some rhinestone buckles I made for the "Bootylicious" video.

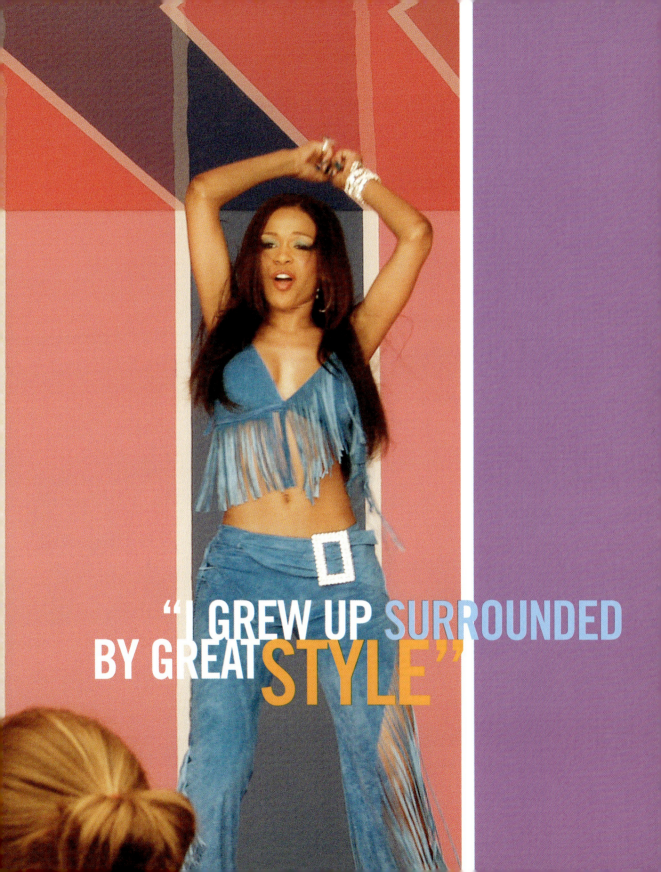

"I GREW UP SURROUNDED BY GREAT STYLE"

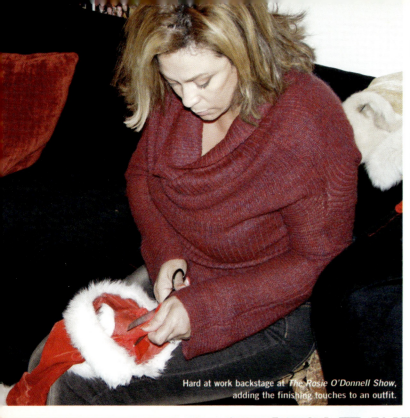

Hard at work backstage at *The Rosie O'Donnell Show*, adding the finishing touches to an outfit.

"i started designing clothing for destiny's child out of sheer necessity"

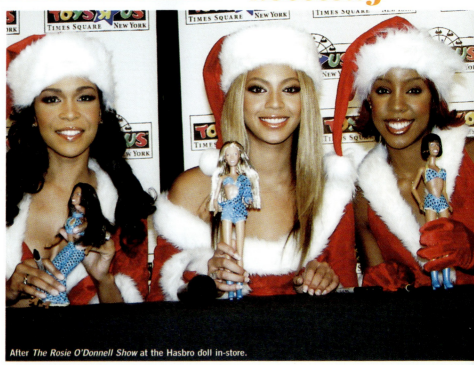

After *The Rosie O'Donnell Show* at the Hasbro doll in-store.

I grew up surrounded by great style and that's as good as any education you get at fashion school. My mama was a seamstress and was always hip to the latest styles. She could knock off anything and made all my clothes. She sewed completely freehand—never used a pattern in her life. Because of her I've always had an eye for fashion and have been handy with a needle and thread. I was the youngest of seven children, so I was pretty much raised as an only child, and I became Mama's chief helper when it came to making clothes and home-decorating projects. Daddy made a living as a longshoreman, and he was slightly deaf, which only allowed him to do certain kinds of work. It was the fifties and work was hard to come by—especially for a black man down in Galveston, Texas, where I was born. So Mama and I worked on our household projects ourselves—we painted, built cabinets, redesigned the kitchen.

Mama was forty-four years old when she had me, so the "Why can't you buy my clothes from the store like everyone else?" battle cry was familiar to her because of my older siblings. One day after hearing an earful of my sassin' she sat me down and told me that I shouldn't be so concerned with what other people were wearing, and instead I should appreciate how special one-of-a-kind clothing with hand-smocking and beadwork is. Basically her words went in one ear and out the other back then. The fact that all my clothes were handmade and unique did nothing but frustrate me because I wanted to be like all the other little girls. I didn't see the beauty in what Mama was creating for me with her own two hands until I was much older and became a designer myself.

Years later, when I became a mother, I tried to instill in my girls the value of marching to the beat of your own drum when it comes to style. I would go to discount stores to buy the girls' clothes, then take them home and customize then. A bit of cutting here, some sewing there, and pretty soon I'd have something unique and I hadn't spent much money. Customizing was an activity that was fun for my girls, their friends, and me to do together. To this day, Beyoncé, Solange, and my "daughter" Kelly Rowland all still love to do it.

As the wardrobe stylist and designer for Destiny's Child, I have created the group's signature style statement. Their style wasn't something that anyone could have predicted or planned; it just sort of happened and caught on. I started designing clothing for Destiny's Child out of sheer necessity. In the beginning, no one knew who the group was and other stylists weren't able to capture their individual personalities and translate that into their clothing, so I began doing it.

Beyoncé may be the only one in Destiny's Child related to me by blood, but Kelly has been living with us since she was twelve years old. I am a second mom to her, and Michelle's become part of the family as well. So, instinctively I know how to style them—that's not a skill money or training can buy. Truth be told, it's not really as complicated as many people will have you believe. All it takes is a belief in yourself and a solid idea of the statement that you want to make. It took me a while to really understand this, so I know how intimidating it can be to explore and play with your personal style. At first, I didn't trust my own creativity because I didn't know how others would react to what I designed. I was afraid the fashion community would think my designs weren't professional, sophisticated, or stylish. Once I had the courage to just go on ahead and "do my thing," the reaction was positive and that encouraged me to continue. Pretty soon there was no turning back. I began to disown the concepts "you can't do that," "you don't have the qualifications for that," or my favorite line, "that won't work—it's never been done." Oh, really? Maybe it's my stubborn streak, but whenever people tell me that or even hint at it, I make it my business to prove them wrong.

It's my hope that I can inspire you to get on out there and "do your thing" too. Remember, there are no limitations to your creativity unless you put them on yourself or allow others to put restrictions on you. No matter what, I always try my best. Because I know that if I try and it doesn't work out, at least I had the courage to get out there and give it my best shot—and that's an accomplishment in itself. My daughter Beyoncé taught me that principle. She's a talented singer, songwriter, music producer, and actress, and in the beginning she never received the credit she deserved. Instead, people in the industry tried to pat her on the head and dismiss her because she's young—but she kept on doing what she does and pretty soon people had to give her the respect she was due. Beyoncé just won the Best Pop Songwriter of the Year award given by ASCAP. She is not only the youngest person to ever receive this award, but also the first African American.

I'm blessed to have been surrounded by people along the way who have helped and encouraged me to cultivate my talents. From my mama who taught me to sew, decorate, and cook, to my husband who bought me a house in which I've honed these skills, to my daughters who were never embarrassed (as I once was) to march to the beat of their own drum, and to my talented nephew Johnny Rittenhouse, who was the best undiscovered designer in the world. (He's since passed, may he rest in peace.) Who I am today is a result of my family and my experiences. I'd also be lost without Hyme, who makes my designs a reality, and Ty Hunter, my assistant. All these people inspired me to develop creatively and have the courage to write this book, which shares my style with the world. So from my heart and hands to yours—*enjoy!*

Beyoncé and I at the *Honey* photo shoot.

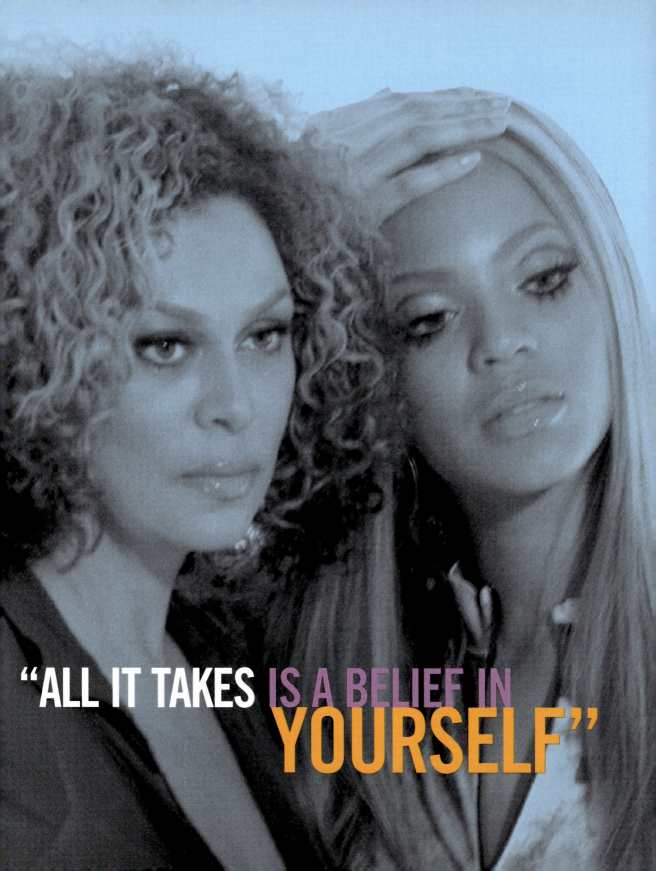

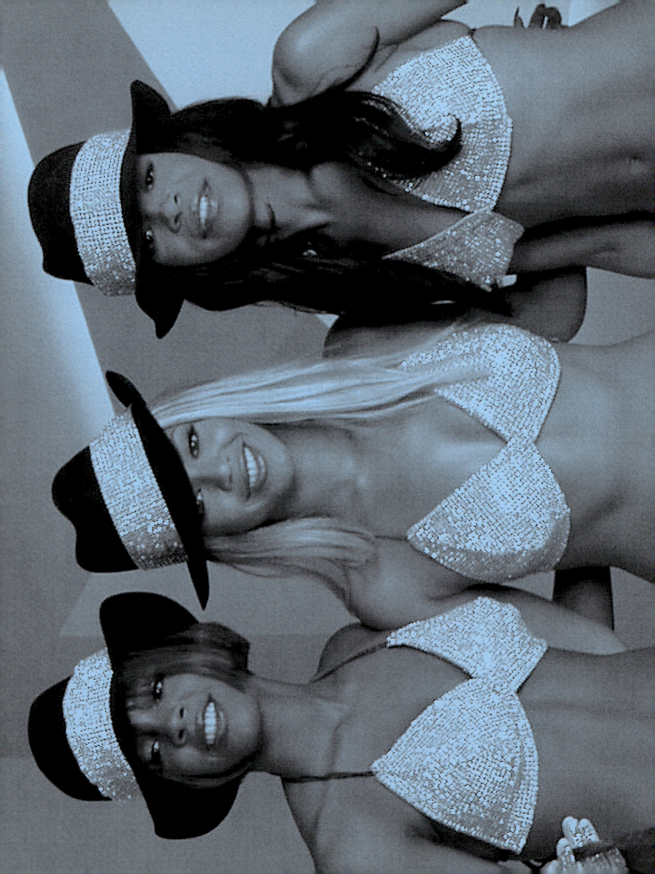

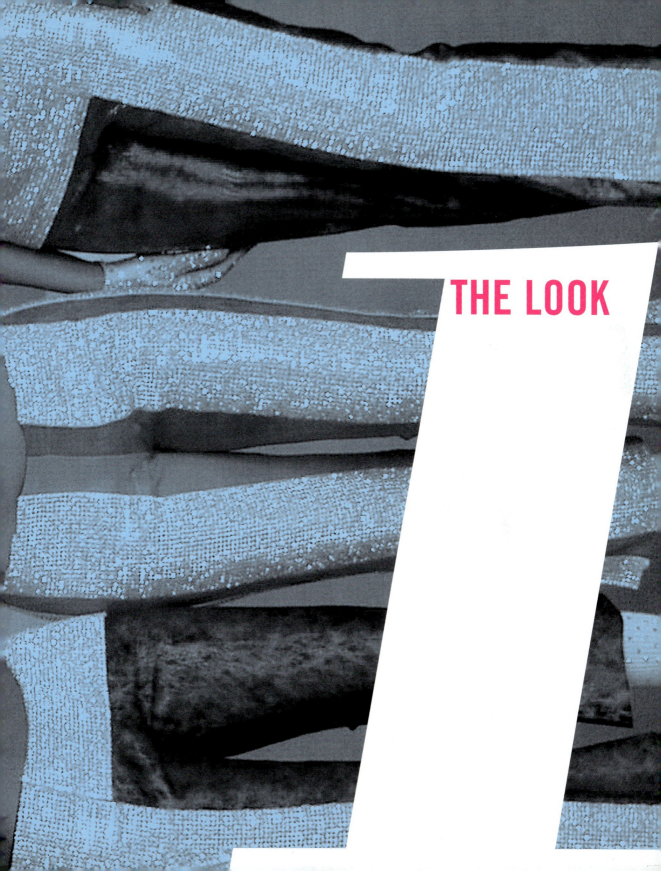

THE LOOK

My first introduction to grown-up fashion came in my twenties. Marvin Gaye's *What's Going On?* album was the soundtrack to my life at that time. Songs like "Inner City Blues (Makes Me Wanna Holler)" captured the spirit of the day for me. Those were times of political changes for the country, and personal changes in the way I saw myself as a woman and as a person of color. The fashion that inspires me when creating the Destiny's Child look is the free and independent spirit of that era. The urban looks of the apple hats that the Jackson 5 would wear to the slinky long dresses that the Supremes wore to the fun and funky colors Sly and the Family Stone rocked have all influenced outfits I've designed for Destiny's Child.

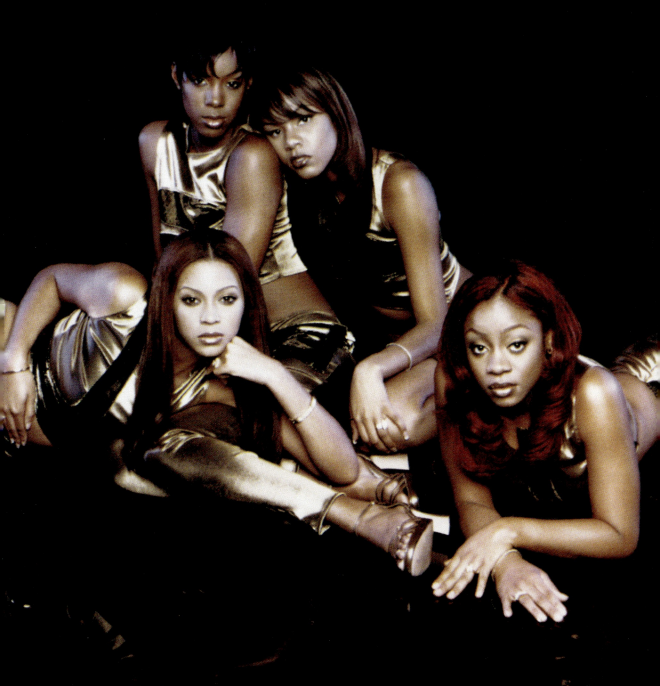

These outfits were created for their self-titled album. I wanted a solid gold look, which was inspired by a James Bond movie I saw on TV.

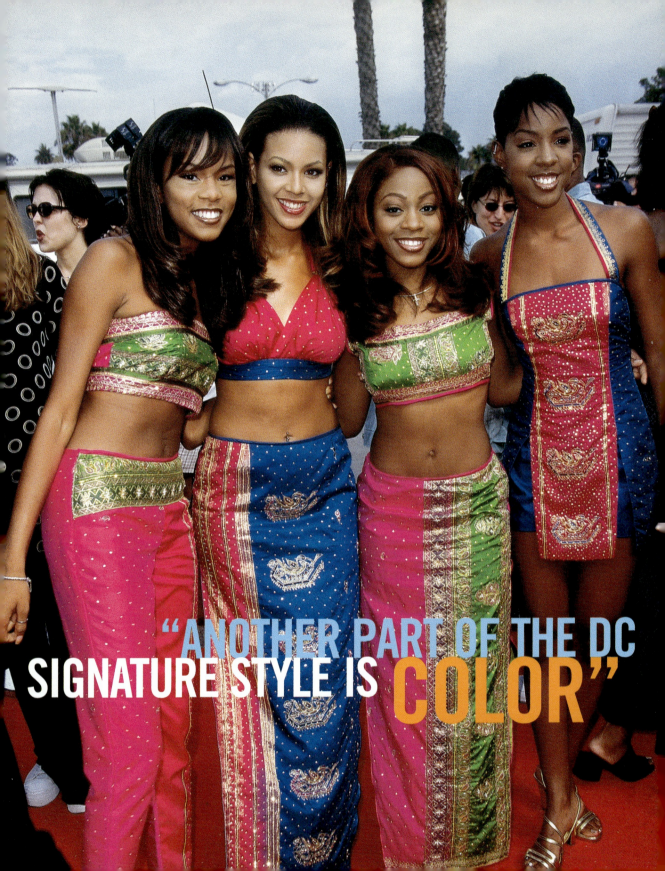

FROM DAY ONE, MATHEW, MY HUSBAND AND DC'S MANAGER, INSISTED THAT THE GIRLS' STYLE BE DIFFERENT THAN ANY OTHER GROUP. IT WAS AN UPHILL BATTLE WITH THE RECORD COMPANY EXECUTIVES BECAUSE THE GENERAL RULE OF THUMB SEEMS TO BE WHEN SOMETHING WORKS THEY DON'T WANT TO CHANGE IT. THEY WANTED DC TO DRESS AND LOOK LIKE ALL THE OTHER GIRL GROUPS THAT WERE OUT THERE. WELL, WHEN THE GIRLS FIRST HIT THE SCENE, IT WAS IN THE MIDDLE OF THE HIP-HOP ERA, WHEN MEN AND WOMEN WERE WEARING BAGGY JEANS AND A REAL CASUAL LOOK. I WENT AGAINST THE GRAIN AND MADE THE CONSCIOUS DECISION THAT I WAS GOING TO BRING BACK THE CLASSIC, SOPHISTICATED LOOK OF MOTOWN, WHEN THE ARTISTS ALL DRESSED UP.

Cher was another inspiration of mine. I remember watching *The Sonny and Cher Show* back in the seventies and Cher's outfits were fabulous. I wanted DC's wardrobe to have a similar glamorous look.

It takes a lot of courage to be willing to separate yourself from the crowd when it comes to fashion—or anything, really. The one thing many people want more than anything is to "fit in" and be like everyone else. My husband said to all of us at the very beginning, "Frankly, I don't give a damn what everyone else in the music industry is doing. Let's do it our way." So we did. The great thing about DC is they make my job so easy, because they don't have the desire to look like everyone else. It's never been a battle to get them to take fashion risks.

I remember one day when Beyoncé was in the fourth grade and she came home from school looking stressed. I asked her what was wrong. She said, "Mama, there's this girl at my school who keeps getting mad at me because she wants me to dress like her and be twins, and I don't want to." I told her to let the girl know that. I figured she'd wait at least until school the next morning, but no, she marched right on over to the phone and called her to let her know she wasn't having any of this "twin" business. Needless to say, Beyoncé was an "independent woman" at an early age, and she found like-minded individuals in Kelly and Michelle.

Another part of the DC signature style is color. I love putting lots of color on the girls. When most people think of dressing stylishly and being sophisticated, they automatically think black clothes. Black is very chic and sexy, but I think you can get just as chic a look with color. It just takes a lot more imagination and effort to do it, but my challenge is always finding new ways to pull it off and make it work. I try hard to make color work for them in a sophisticated way. That's why they wear lots of hand-beaded fabrics, faux fur, and leather. It gives their clothes a fun, carefree, yet stylish look that can be worn to upscale functions like award shows, as well as onstage at concerts and in videos.

These outfits were made from traditional Indian saris.

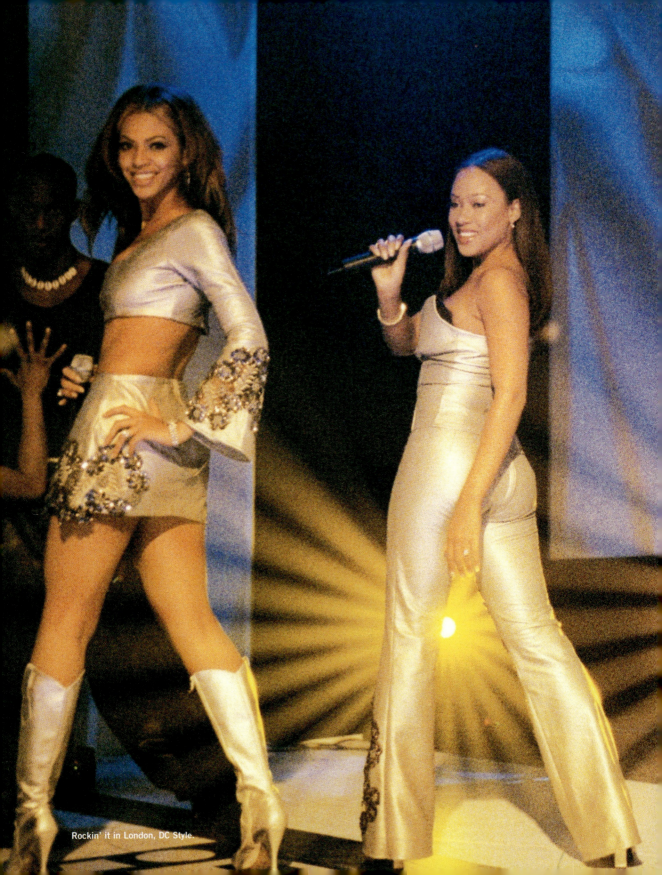
Rockin' it in London, DC Style.

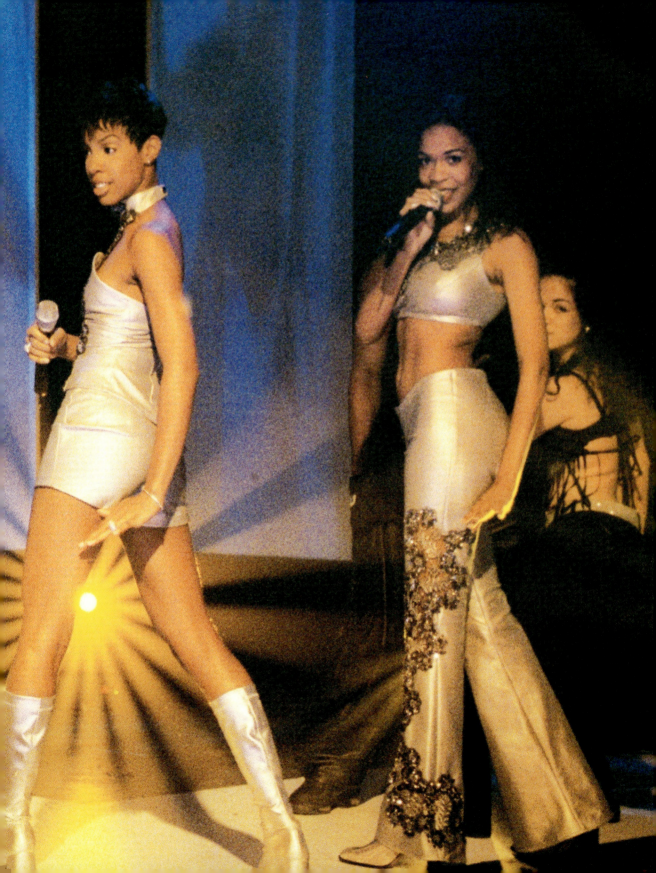

ACHIEVING BOOTYLICIOUSNESS

BEING BOOTYLICIOUS HAS LESS TO DO WITH WHAT OUTFIT YOU'RE ROCKIN' AND MORE TO DO WITH THE FRAME OF MIND AND THE CONFIDENCE YOU EXUDE. THE FRENCH CALL IT *ÊTRE BIEN DANS SA PEAU*, THAT IS, "FEELING HAPPY IN ONE'S OWN SKIN." THE OTHER KEY IS TO BE SEXY WITHOUT LOOKING NASTY, OR "STANK" AS WE CALL IT. PART OF ACHIEVING CLASSY SEXINESS IS TO KNOW YOUR BODY TYPE AND WEAR CLOTHES THAT WORK BEST FOR YOUR SHAPE. SEX APPEAL SHOULD BE SOMETHING THAT'S IMPLIED, NOT STATED. THAT'S WHAT THE "BOOTYLICIOUS" PHILOSOPHY IS ALL ABOUT. THERE'S A SONG BEYONCÉ WROTE, WHICH IS ON DC'S *SURVIVOR* ALBUM, CALLED "NASTY GIRL" THAT ADDRESSES THE ISSUE OF DRESSING WITH SOME PERSONAL INTEGRITY. I GET A LOT OF GREAT FEEDBACK FROM PARENTS AND YOUNG GIRLS ABOUT THE CLOTHES THAT DC WEARS. I'VE FOUND THAT TEENAGE GIRLS (AND THEIR PARENTS) APPRECIATE THE FACT THAT I MAKE BEYONCÉ, KELLY, AND MICHELLE LOOK HOT WITHOUT SEXUALIZING THEM. SINCE I AM BOTH A MOTHER AND A STYLIST, I'VE MADE THE CONSCIOUS EFFORT TO MAKE SURE THE DC WARDROBE IS EYE-CATCHING WITHOUT HAVING THE GIRLS OUT THERE HALF NAKED OR IN CLOTHES THAT ARE ILL-FITTING OR TOO TIGHT—WE CALL THAT LOOK "HOOCHIE. REGARDLESS OF HOW MANY HATS I WEAR, I'M MOM FIRST, AND I WILL NEVER HAVE THE LADIES LOOKING CHEAP. TRUST ME, WE GET ALL KINDS OF PRESSURE FROM MAGAZINES WHO WANT TO BE THE FIRST TO PUT DC ON THEIR COVERS IN BIKINIS, BUT WE DON'T GO THERE.

I grew up in the seventies and wore low hip-huggers and belly-bearing tops. I see nothing vulgar about wearing midriff tops, if your stomach is toned, or shorts (not too short), if you have the legs for them. It's fashion. It's fun. And if you've got it, flaunt it. If people think it's sexy, fine. But I don't believe that clothes alone make a person sexy. Kelly said it best when someone once asked her about sex appeal. She said, "Sexiness comes from within. It's not about how short your skirt is or how much skin you show. It's about being confident and letting that confidence out." When you achieve that—that's when you're truly bootylicious.

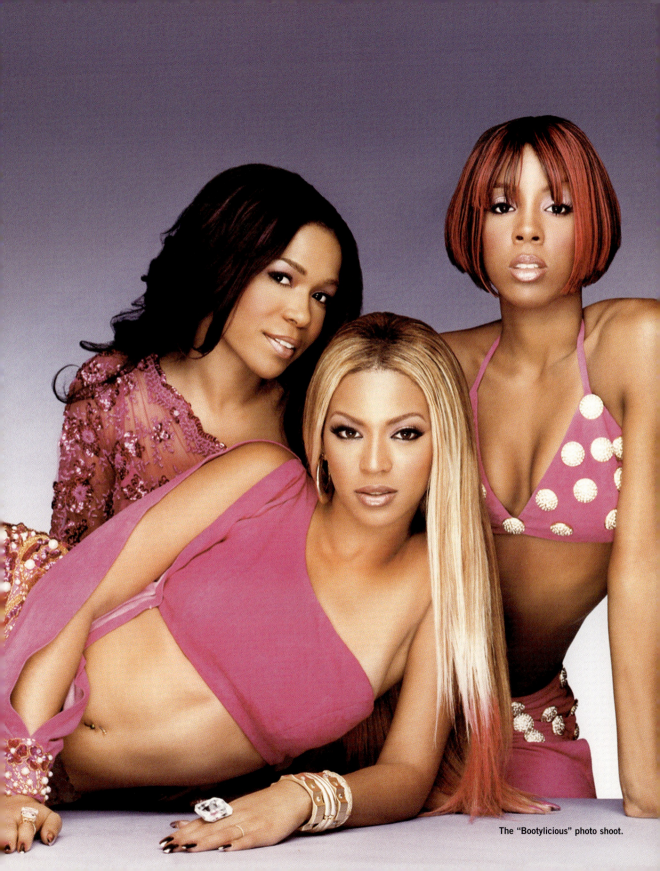

The "Bootylicious" photo shoot.

The Right Fit

BEYONCÉ, KELLY, AND MICHELLE ARE ALL VERY DIFFERENT FROM ONE ANOTHER, AND THEY ARE ALL BEAUTIFUL. BEYONCÉ WITH HER SIGNATURE BLOND HAIR AND HEALTHY CURVES, KELLY WITH HER RED HAIR AND SLINKY BODY, AND MICHELLE WITH HER LONG, DARK HAIR AND SLIM YET WOMANLY FIGURE REPRESENT THREE DIFFERENT BODY TYPES FOR PEOPLE TO RELATE TO. THEY'VE BECOME STYLE ROLE MODELS AND THEY TAKE THAT VERY SERIOUSLY. THEY ARE VERY AWARE THAT WHAT THEY WEAR AND HOW THEY PORTRAY THEIR BODY IMAGE IS HEAVILY WATCHED BY MILLIONS OF PEOPLE. IT'S HARD SOMETIMES BECAUSE THEY HAVE DAYS LIKE EVERYONE ELSE WHEN THEY ARE BLOATED, OUT OF SHAPE, AND HAVE COMPLEXION PROBLEMS.

All of us have aspects of our bodies that we are uncomfortable with. It doesn't matter if you are a little thicker than you'd like to be in some places or a little skinnier than you'd like to be in others—we all have areas we like to camouflage. On the flip side, there are parts of our bodies that we can look at in the mirror and say, "Yeah, girl, you got it goin' on!" One of the keys to having all-over body satisfaction when you get dressed is simply dressing right for your body type. Clothes, if properly worn and proportioned, can create illusions you never thought were possible. Trust me, with the right fit anybody can look bootylicious.

I dress each of the DC ladies in clothes that flatter her particular figure. I think the whole idea of women aspiring to be thin or having a certain bust size is ridiculous. The amount of time and energy women spend hating parts of their bodies because a fashion magazine says they ought to is wrong. Being sexy is knowing how to work the jelly the good Lord gave you. You have a bootylicious booty and healthy hips? Work it, chile. Beyoncé does! So you don't like your legs? It ain't no thing. Neither does Michelle, so she prefers to wear pants. Kelly's one of those women who has come to terms with her body and loves it now. She used to wish she was thicker and more voluptuous because she would get teased about being so darn skinny. Now she works what she's got and is quite happy. Beyoncé, Kelly, and Michelle are great models for demonstrating how to use proportion to look your best.

"beyoncé, kelly, and michelle are all very different from one another, and they are all beautiful"

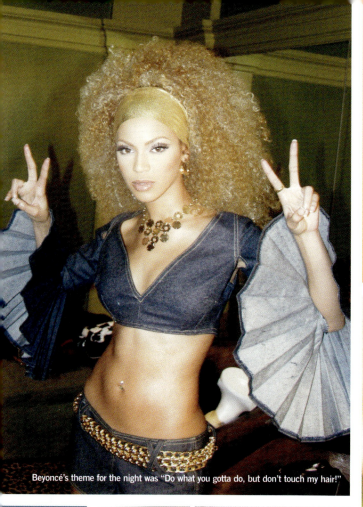

Beyoncé's theme for the night was "Do what you gotta do, but don't touch my hair!"

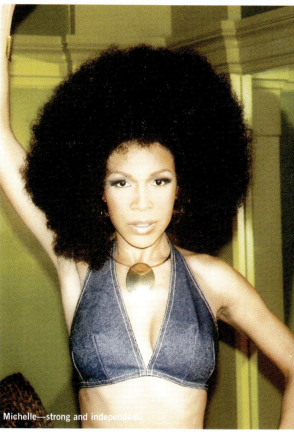

Michelle—strong and independent.

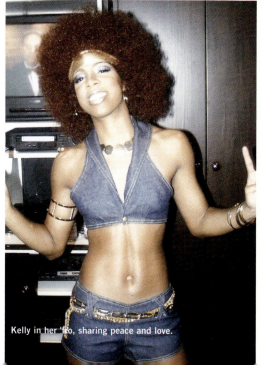

Kelly in her 'fro, sharing peace and love.

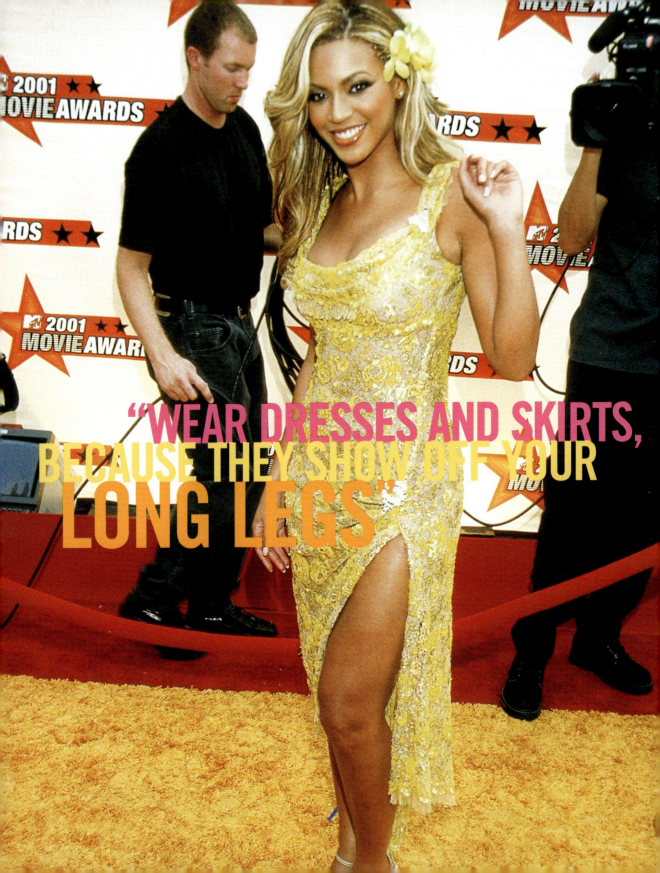

What to Wear?

IF YOU'RE BUILT LIKE BEYONCÉ THEN YOU'RE A VERY CURVY GIRL WITH AMPLE HIPS AND THIGHS, A TINY WAIST, A LONG TORSO, AND GREAT LEGS. WOMEN WHO ARE SHAPED LIKE THIS LOOK BEST IN DRESSES. THE FOLLOWING CLOTHES LOOK BEST ON YOU IF YOU SHARE HER BODY TYPE:

- Wear dresses and skirts, because they show off your long legs. If you want to go for *really* short skirts, wear shorts under them that are the same color as the skirt.

- Dresses should be fitted from the bust to the waist and flare slightly at the hips to create an even proportion between your slim upper body and curvy lower body.

- Wear A-line skirts. They should be made of a solid, heavy fabric.

- To focus attention on your small waist and lean upper body, either wear midriff tops or very long tops, but avoid ones that hit at the waist—they cut you in half.

- Avoid severe bell-bottoms or wide straight pants. These silhouettes tend to weigh you down and don't accentuate your long legs.

IF HAVE A BODY LIKE KELLY, LEAN WITH BROAD SHOULDERS, A TINY WAIST, AND NARROW HIPS, YOU PROBABLY GOT TEASED WHEN YOU WERE YOUNGER FOR BEING SKINNY AND NOT HAVING BOOTY—JUST LIKE SHE DID. MY, HOW THINGS HAVE CHANGED! THESE DAYS SHE COULD WEAR A GARBAGE BAG AND LOOK GOOD. WOMEN WHO HAVE AN EVENLY PROPORTIONED BODY CAN EXPERIMENT WITH UNIQUE OR "OUT THERE" FASHION STYLES. IF YOU HAVE A BODY LIKE KELLY'S, THEN THE FOLLOWING CLOTHES LOOK GREAT ON YOU:

- All types of pants look good, particularly ones that are slim-fitting through the leg.

- Miniskirts are a must for showing off your long legs. Even if you're not typically a miniskirt girl, you owe it to yourself to have one in your wardrobe for those days you're feeling daring.

- Wear shirts that show off your arms.

- Exotic neck jewelry like antique chokers and amulet necklaces look great on you.

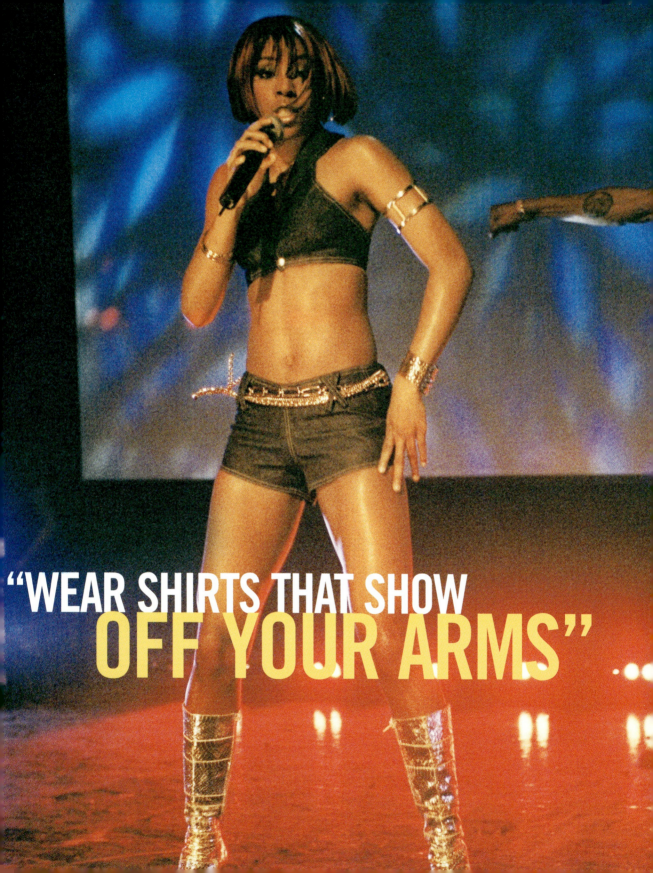

MICHELLE HAS BROAD SHOULDERS, A SHORT TORSO, AND LONG LEGS. SHE'S SLIM AND CURVY, WHICH IS NOT VERY COMMON. SHE HAPPENS TO HAVE A THING ABOUT HER LEGS. SHE'S SAID THAT SHE THINKS HER LEGS LOOK LIKE UPSIDE-DOWN BASEBALL BATS. THEY DON'T, BUT SINCE SHE FEELS MORE COMFORTABLE IN PANTS, I ACCOMMODATE HER. IF YOUR BODY LOOKS LIKE MICHELLE'S, HERE ARE SOME THINGS THAT YOU SHOULD KEEP IN MIND WHEN PLANNING YOUR WARDROBE:

- Stick to pants that fall below your belly button. High-waisted pants will make your torso look shorter.

- Three-quarter-length skirts look good on you.

- Halter tops that tie around the neck look great because they show off your shoulders.

- Slim, form-fitting dresses that cling to your waist and hips and fall below the knee show off your curves nicely.

- Avoid wearing shoulder pads. Since you have broad shoulders, there's no reason to.

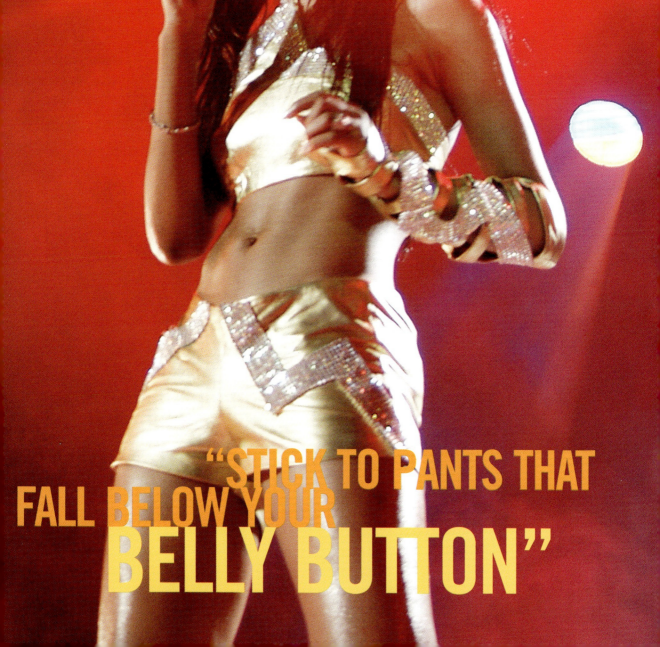

IT'S IN THE JEANS

I BELIEVE THAT THE BEST THING A GIRL CAN DO FOR HERSELF IS TO GET A PAIR OF JEANS THAT FIT HER BODY PERFECTLY—ONES THAT DON'T MAKE YOUR BUTT LOOK FLAT OR AREN'T TOTALLY UNFLATTERING. A GREAT-FITTING PAIR OF JEANS CAN BE HARD TO FIND, BUT ONCE YOU FIND THEM THEY CAN QUICKLY BECOME YOUR FAVORITE ARTICLE OF CLOTHING. NOT TOO TIGHT, NOT TOO SAGGY, THAT EVER ELUSIVE "JUST RIGHT" FIT IS A MUST.

Kelly and Michelle can wear most pants and jeans right off the rack, and the fit is perfect. Beyoncé has classic womanly curves. She's built like that old Commodores song "Brick House." Like a lot of sistas, she has ample booty and a small waist. So her jeans need to be very low-waisted. It's always been worth it to buy her jeans one size too big and have them cut down to fit her. The difference in the fit is remarkable. Try it and see if it works for you.

It's totally worth making the investment of taking a pair of jeans to a good tailor to have them fitted to you body. The price of tailoring jeans varies. I've paid anywhere from fifteen to seventy-five dollars, so shop around. Jeans are something you can wear over and over each day with different tops so you'll definitely get your money's worth.

Simple accessories, like belts, can jazz up a basic jeans and halter top outfit. Check out the girls' customized jeans.

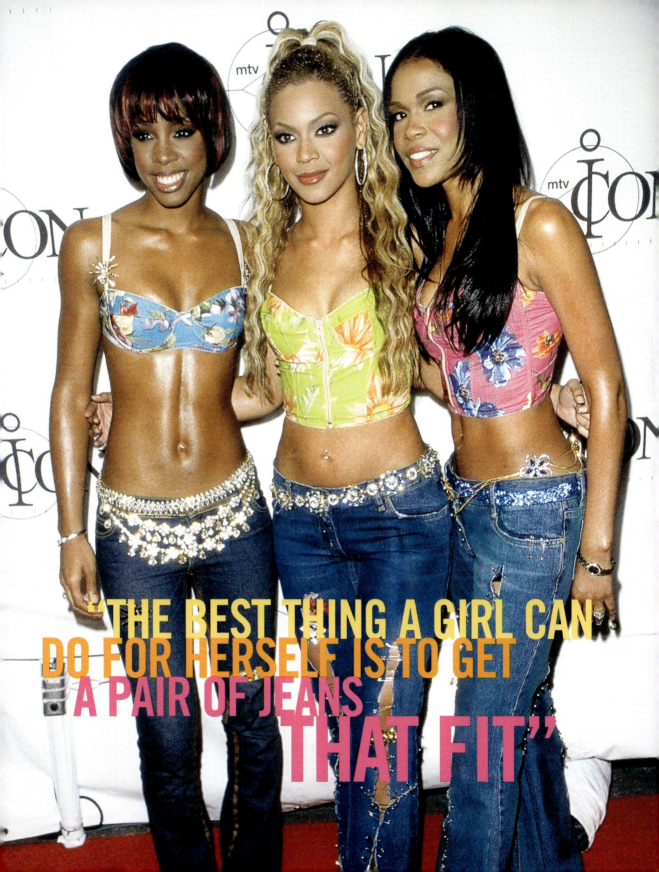

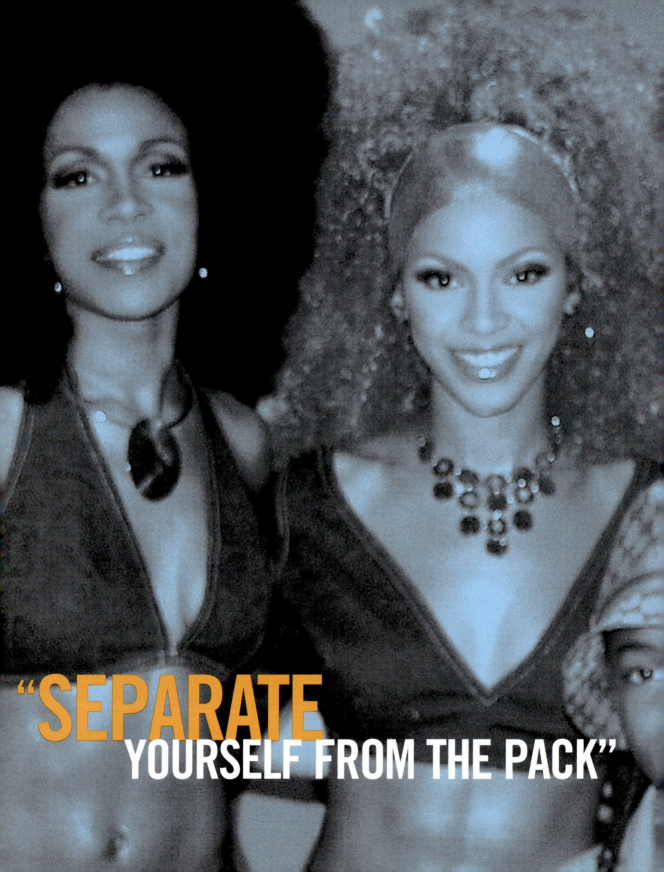

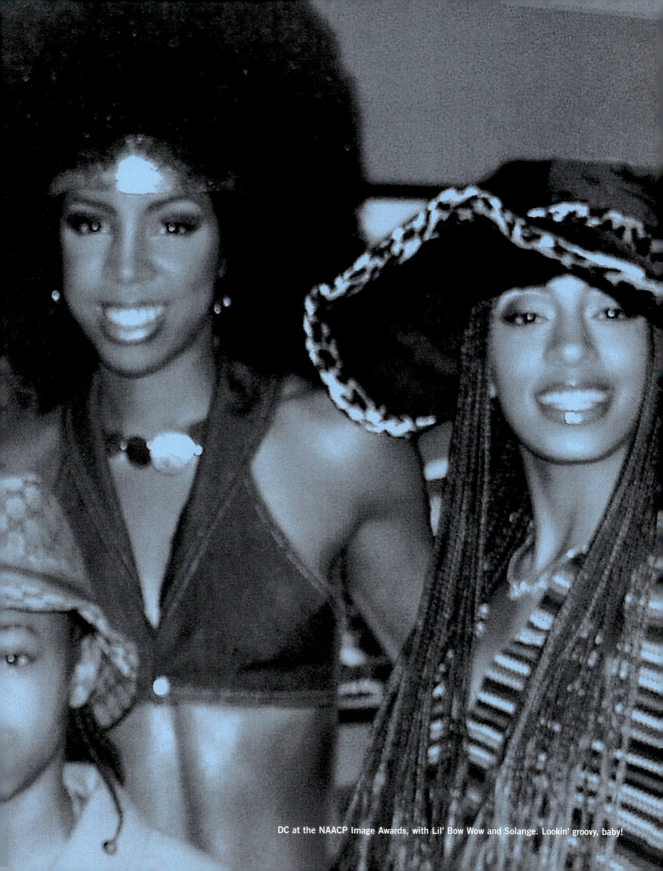

DC at the NAACP Image Awards, with Lil' Bow Wow and Solange. Lookin' groovy, baby!

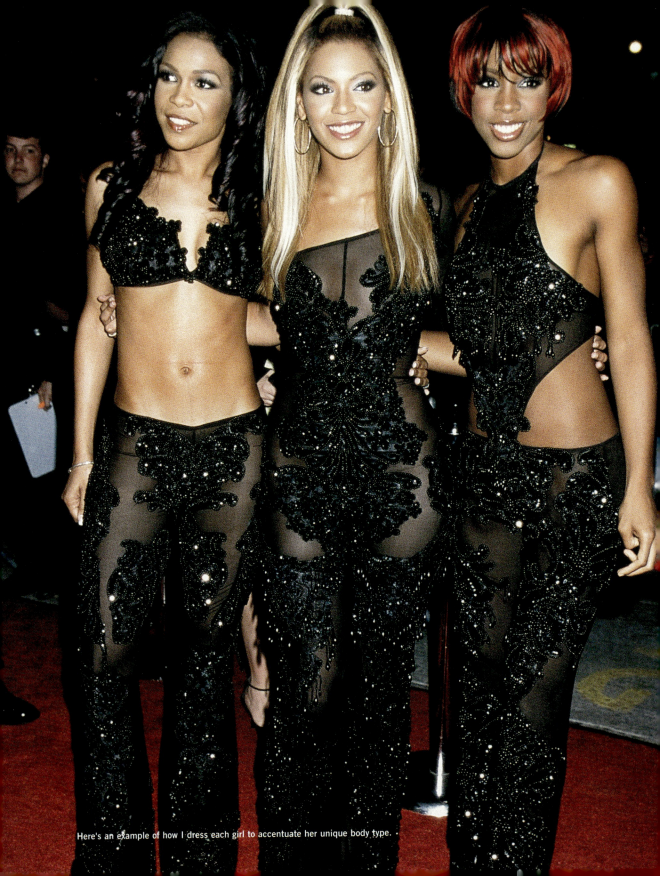

Here's an example of how I dress each girl to accentuate her unique body type.

HEY, GIRLFRIEND! A WORD OF CAUTION

When you see someone onstage, in a magazine, or in a video wearing an outfit you love, before hijacking their look, ask yourself, "Is it appropriate for my real life?" Entertainers are in show business—they often wear avant-garde and sometimes sexy outfits in the same way a surgeon wears gloves or an attorney wears a suit. If you're a student or work in an office, there's no reason to dress like the ultimate video vixen. That's not hot. There's a time and place for everything. Beyoncé, Kelly, and Michelle don't wear their Destiny's Child outfits when they aren't performing. There's a fine line between bootylicious and hootchylicious.

BOOTYLICIOUS

1. SEPARATING YOURSELF FROM THE PACK WHEN IT COMES TO FASHION—TRYING NEW THINGS.
2. EXPERIMENTING WITH COLORFUL CLOTHES.
3. LOOKING TO THE STYLE ICONS OF THE PAST FOR INSPIRATION.
4. RESPECTING THE LINE BETWEEN SEXY/CLASSY AND NASTY/TRASHY.
5. UNDERSTANDING PROPORTION. IF YOU WEAR A BIKINI OR CROP TOP, WEAR A LONG SKIRT OR LOW-SLUNG PANTS. IF YOU WEAR A SHORT SKIRT OR HOT PANTS, WEAR A LONG TOP. OTHERWISE YOU LOOK LIKE YOU'RE WALKING AROUND HALF NAKED.

VERSUS

HOOTCHYLICIOUS

1. COPYING ALL THE LATEST FADS AND WORRYING ABOUT WHAT OTHER PEOPLE ARE DOING STYLE-WISE.
2. WEARING CLOTHES THAT ARE TOO TIGHT OR NOT FLATTERING TO YOUR BODY TYPE.
3. HAVING YOUR BOOTY HANGING OUT OF TOO SHORT MINISKIRTS OR HOT PANTS.
4. UNDIES SHOWING FROM THE TOP OF LOW-SLUNG PANTS.
5. BOOBS HANGING OUT FROM UNDER SHORT BIKINI TOPS OR HALTER TOPS.

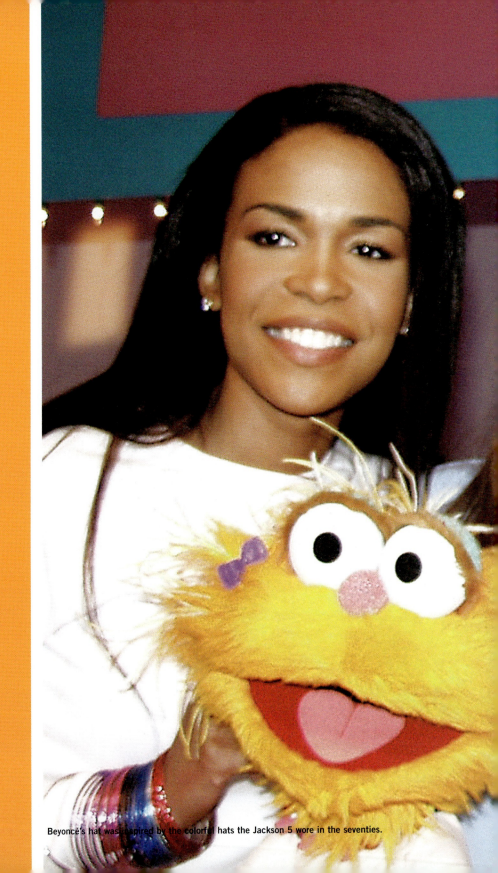

Beyoncé's hat was inspired by the colorful hats the Jackson 5 wore in the seventies.

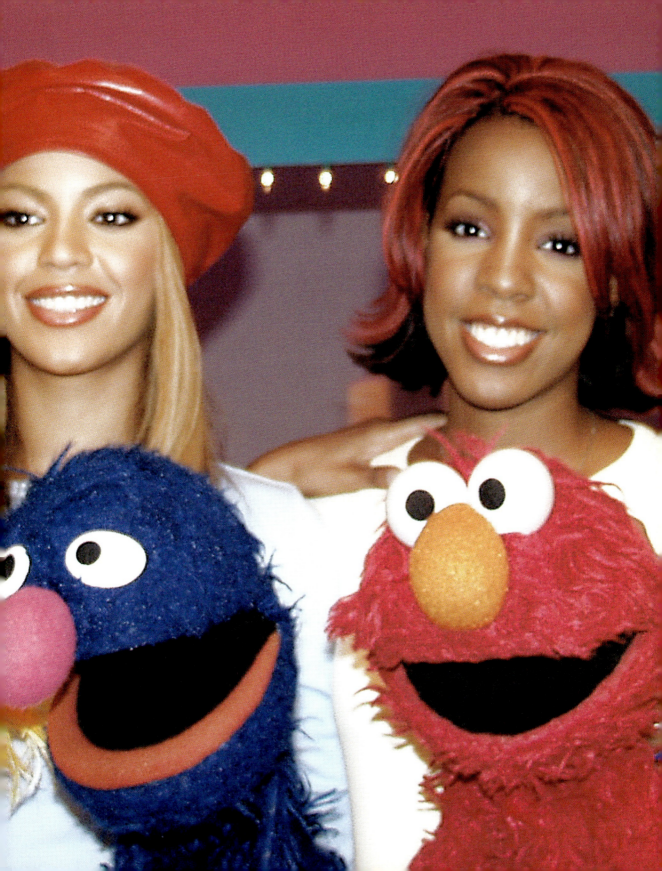

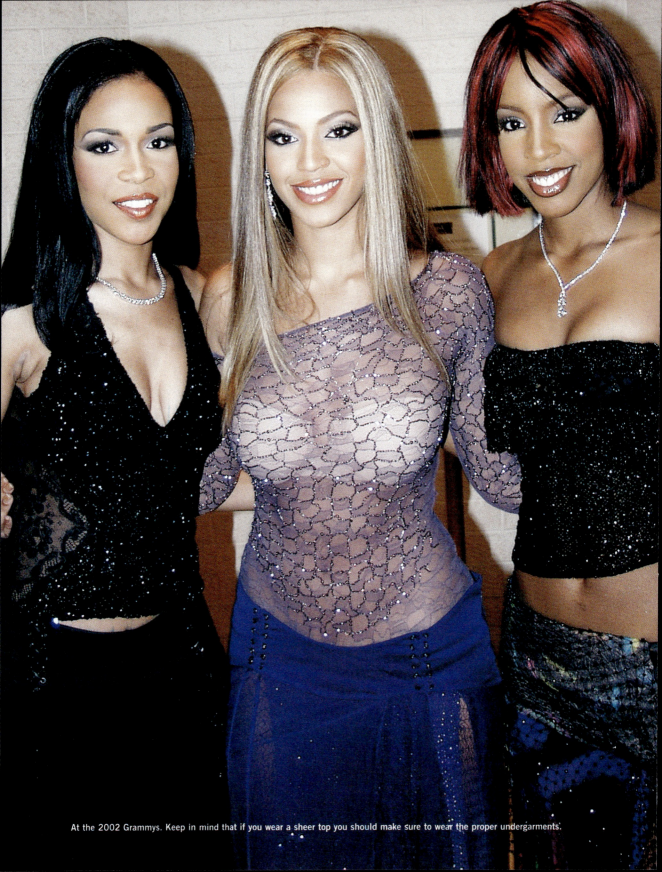

At the 2002 Grammys. Keep in mind that if you wear a sheer top you should make sure to wear the proper undergarments.

A SOLID FOUNDATION

IF THERE'S ONE THING I'VE LEARNED IN THIS BUSINESS IT'S THAT THERE'S A REASON UNDERWEAR IS CALLED A "FOUNDATION GARMENT." WHEN IT COMES DOWN TO IT, THE RIGHT UNDERWEAR CAN MAKE OR BREAK AN OUTFIT. WEARING INCORRECT UNDERWEAR FOR YOUR OUTFIT IS LIKE A PAINTER TRYING TO PAINT ON BUMPY OR BADLY STRETCHED CANVAS. A LOT OF DC'S ULTRASLEEK LOOKS WOULD NEVER WORK IF THE PROPER UNDERWEAR WASN'T IN PLACE. AFTER ALL, PANTIES THAT ARE TOO HIGH-WAISTED AND PEEK OUT FROM THE TOPS OF PANTS MAY WORK FOR RAP ARTISTS, BUT FOR LADIES I DON'T THINK IT'S CUTE. A BRA THAT GIVES AN UNFLATTERING SHAPE TO YOUR BUSTLINE OR PEEKS OUT FROM UNDER YOUR CLOTHES DOESN'T HELP AN OUTFIT LOOK GOOD EITHER.

When shopping for underwear or getting dressed, keep in mind the outfit you plan on wearing. If the outfit is semitransparent, wear a bra that matches your skin tone. Wear flesh-colored undies under light-colored clothes and black undies under dark-colored clothing. Seamless bras provide a more natural look for most form-fitting clothes, and low-waisted panties should be worn when wearing low-slung jeans or hip-hugging pants.

Quick Tips for Foundation Bug A Boos

If you can't find flesh-colored underwear that matches your skin tone, you can make your own by dyeing white underwear. Mix tan and brown Rit dye. Start with the tan dye and add brown to it until the color matches your skin tone—the brown dye cuts the green tone in the tan dye. Then dip plain white underwear in the solution; inexpensive ones made of a satiny material work well. If you dye four pairs of panties and four bras you've got enough skin-toned underwear to wear under all of your outfits.

Or you can try "tacking" as a shortcut. Tacking is lightly sewing material onto something else in long stitches, just so the fabric stays in place. Before I started dyeing underwear to match the girls' skin tone, I'd go buy pantyhose that matched their skin color. I'd get the thickest pantyhose in the biggest size I could find and cut it to fit, then "tack" it onto their bra cups. This is a temporary solution for a problem that needs to be solved quickly, like if you're going out for the evening and you put on your top only to discover the bra is showing through.

Trying the same top with a skirt, shorts, and long pants. It's appropriate for each of the girls' body types.

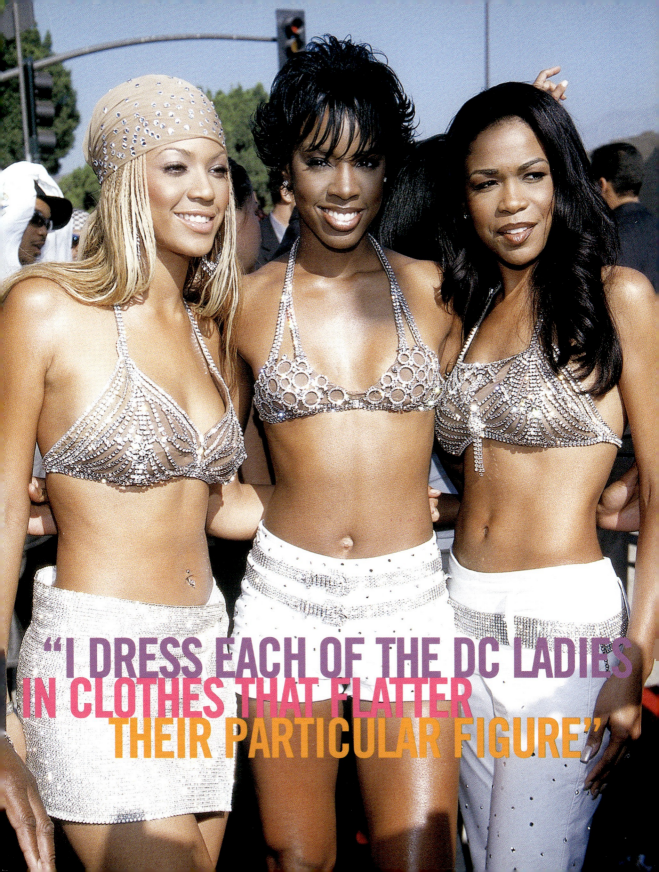

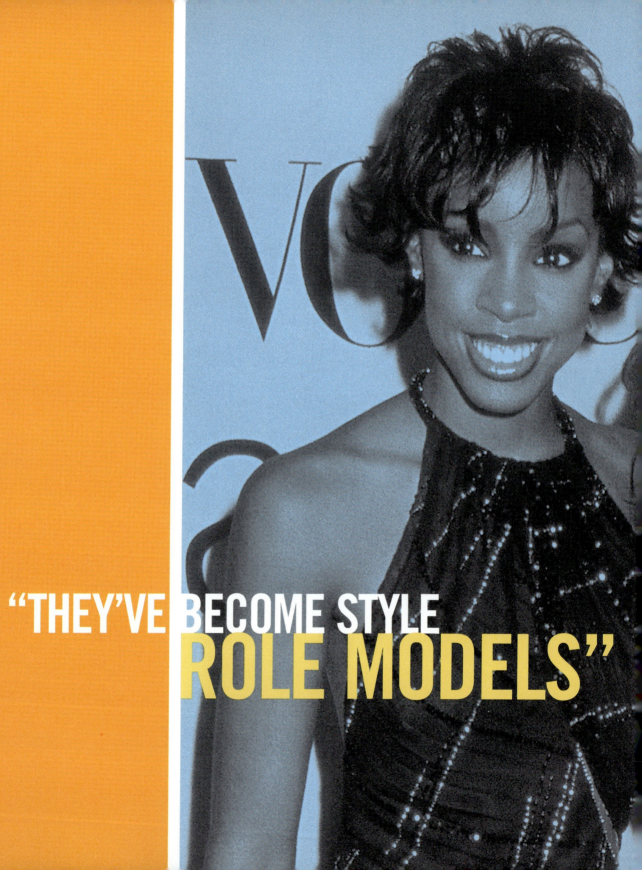

"THEY'VE BECOME STYLE ROLE MODELS"

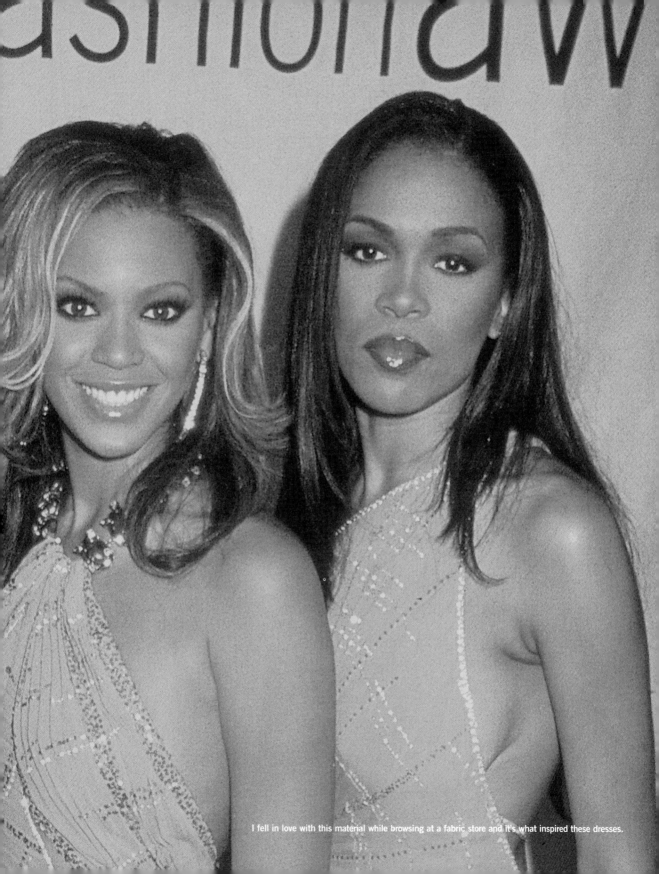

I fell in love with this material while browsing at a fabric store and it's what inspired these dresses.

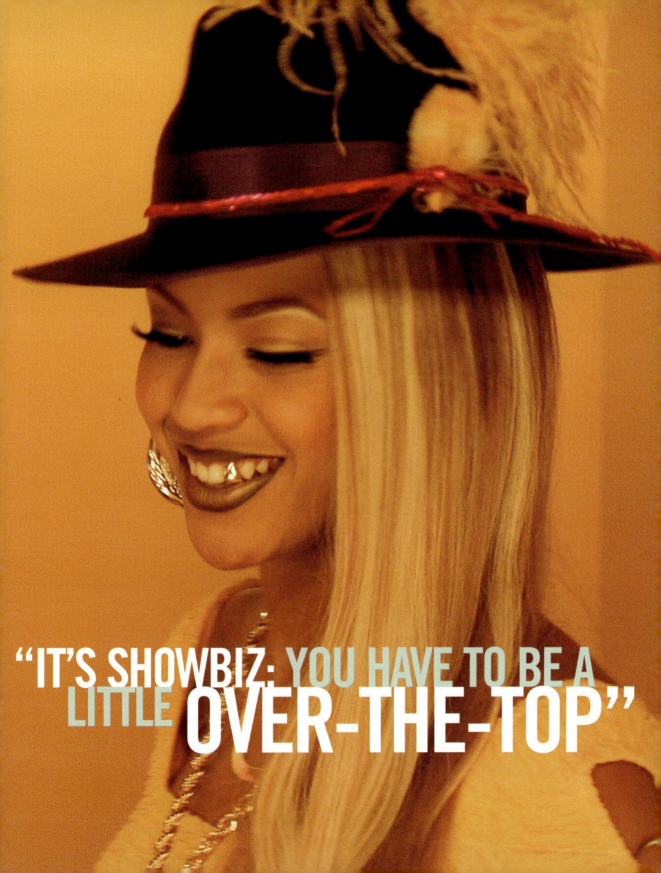

"IT'S SHOWBIZ: YOU HAVE TO BE A LITTLE OVER-THE-TOP"

ACCESSORIZING

IN THE DAYS BEFORE DESTINY'S CHILD SOLD MILLIONS OF RECORDS, THE WARDROBE BUDGET WAS TIGHT—BEYOND TIGHT. IT WAS THEN THAT I DISCOVERED THE POWER OF ACCESSORIES. ACCESSORIES CAN MAKE A REALLY INEXPENSIVE OUTFIT LOOK LIKE A DESIGNER ORIGINAL. IF YOU LOOK AT EARLY DC VIDEOS LIKE "BUG A BOO," YOU CAN SEE HOW I USED HATS AND BIG JEWELRY TO JAZZ UP SOME AVERAGE-LOOKING OUTFITS. EVEN IN LATER VIDEOS LIKE THE ONE FOR "BOOTYLICIOUS," WHICH WAS ONE OF THEIR MOST EXPENSIVE, I USED LOTS OF BIG, FUN ACCESSORIES LIKE GOLD CHAINS, HATS, AND FEATHERS ON ONE OF THEIR WARDROBE CHANGES TO ADD TO THAT GHETTO FABULOUS FEEL. THESE YELLOW OUTFITS WERE INSPIRED BY FLEA MARKET TRENDY CLOTHES—IT WAS SO MUCH FUN.

The thing I love most about accessories is that they can be cheap and versatile. For instance, a twelve-dollar chain belt can also work as a bracelet. Just wrap it around your wrist a few times and close the clasp. It's easy and you can achieve the look of having a lot of bracelets without having to spend money on them individually. Remember, one really cool piece to dress up an outfit is always much better than having too many things going on. When I get the girls ready for videos or performances, I always overaccessorize them. After all, it's showbiz; you have to be a little over-the-top. On their days off the girls love accessories, but they don't go overboard with them.

Check out that gold tooth.

BOOTYLICIOUS ACCESSORIES CHECKLIST

1. Interesting necklaces. Cool chokers, intricate antique necklaces, and big chunky amulet necklaces can add pizzazz to any outfit. They can be found at really reasonable prices in the juniors section in department stores or at inexpensive costume jewelry chain stores like Claire's boutique. 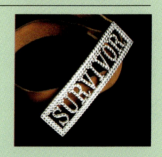 *2. Fun belts.* Skinny chain belts and thick chunky belts add drama to an outfit and are an easy way to add a little oomph. I use them all the time when an outfit needs a pick-me-up. Vintage belts are great and inexpensive too. *3. Bracelets.* I like dressing up bare arms with thick bracelets. Bracelets are popular accessories with all three ladies. They've all bought each other diamond bracelets as gifts. *4. Pins.* In the "Bootylicious" video I attached rhinestone buckles to the belts and chokers of the blue outfits DC wore. Pins can really add drama to an outfit. *5. Belly chains.* Don't be afraid of belly chains if you don't like your belly. They are a very versatile addition to any wardrobe and can be worn either as belts or around your neck as a necklace. I've used them in a few photo shoots that way. Beyoncé loves belly chains so much that Mathew bought her a diamond one as a gift.

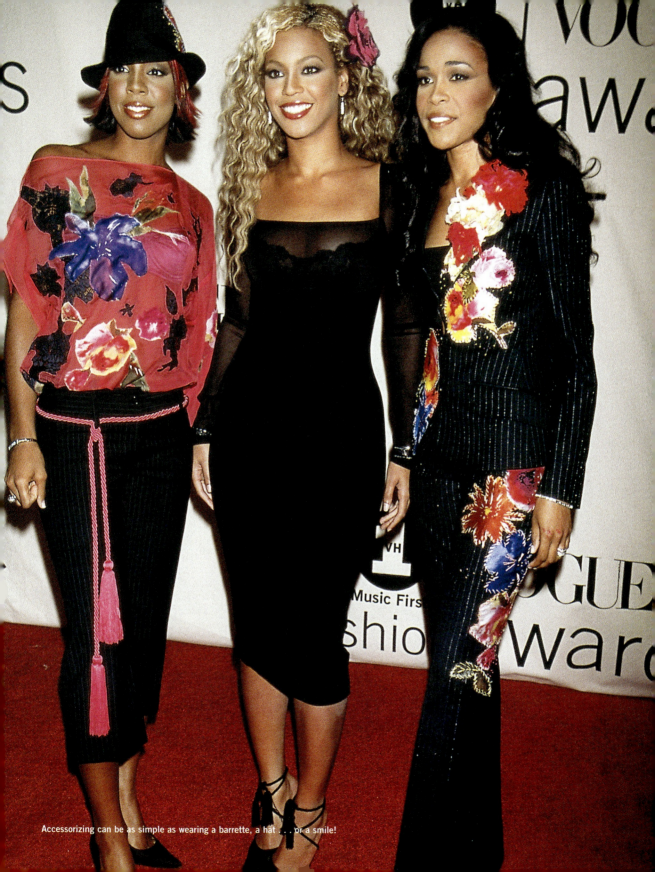
Accessorizing can be as simple as wearing a barrette, a hat . . . or a smile!

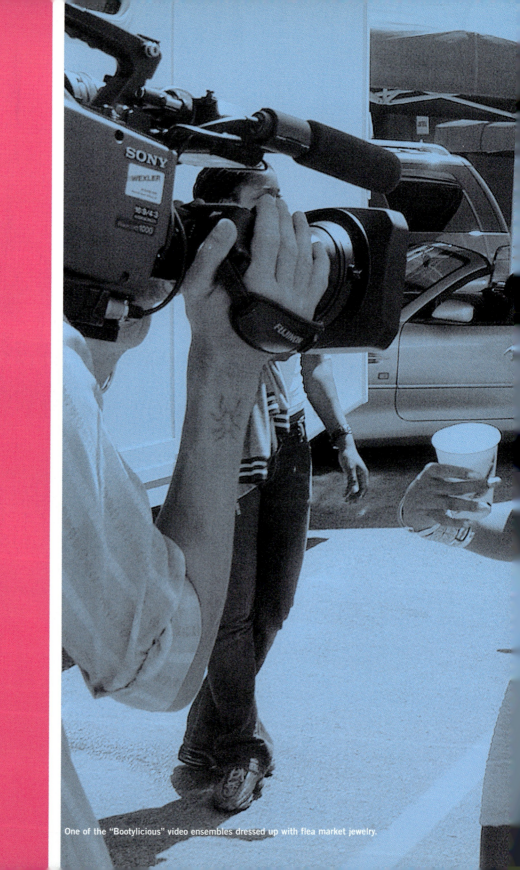
One of the "Bootylicious" video ensembles dressed up with flea market jewelry.

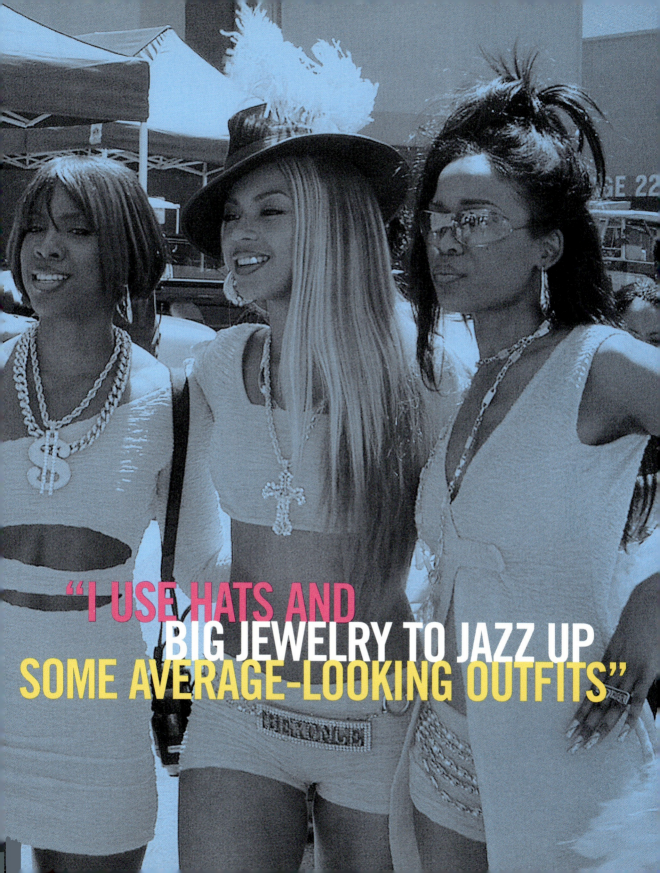

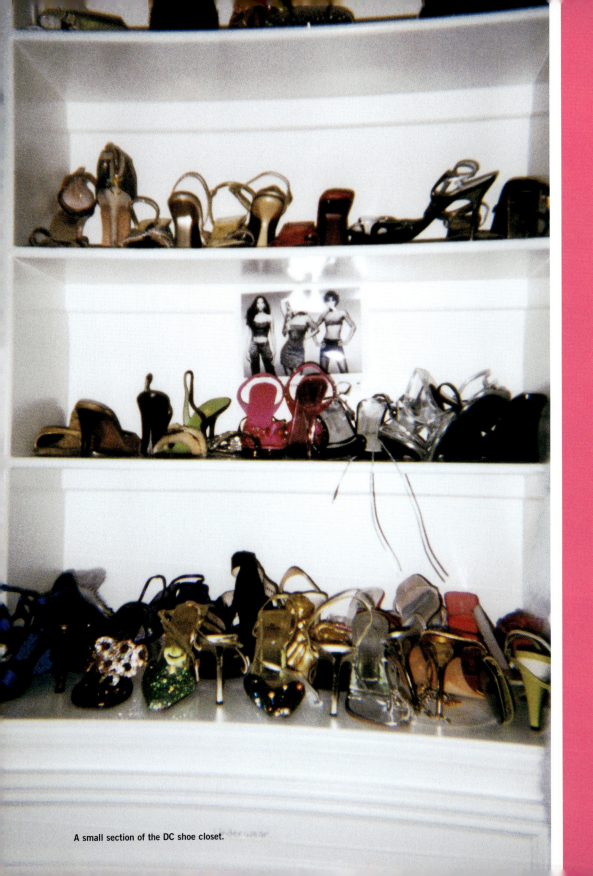

A small section of the DC shoe closet.

SHOES

WHEN I WAS IN MY EARLY TWENTIES, I PURCHASED A PAIR OF WHITE THIGH-HIGH BOOTS FROM A STORE IN MY HOMETOWN. I REMEMBER THEY COST ME NEARLY TWO HUNDRED DOLLARS, AND BACK THEN THAT WAS *REALLY* A LOT OF MONEY FOR A PAIR OF BOOTS. I HAD THOSE THINGS ON LAYAWAY FOR MORE THAN SIX MONTHS. WHEN I FINALLY PAID FOR THEM, I WORE THE HECK OUT OF THEM. I EVEN MADE OUTFITS FOR THE SOLE PURPOSE OF HAVING SOMETHING TO WEAR WITH THE BOOTS.

A lot of women have a weakness for shoes, and the women of DC are no exception. Luckily, they all happen to wear the same shoe size, size 9, so they are always trading shoes with one another. Thank goodness they love high heels, because heels are the staple of the DC look. Whether it's the boots they wore during MTV's 2001 Total Request Live Tour, which I spray-painted gold and glued rhinestones to the heels of, or the death-defying gold stilettos the girls worked on the VH-1 "Divas Live" concert, their shoes are always high and fierce.

I believe high heels can be a girl's best friend. They create an incredible illusion by giving skinny legs curves and streamlining heavier legs. In heels, your upper body becomes straight, and you're instantly taller. I'm always in high heels, even when I'm dressing casual. While other people wear Keds or tennis shoes, I'll throw on a pair of high-heeled mules. I'm so accustomed to heels that I don't feel like myself without them on, and my feet are so used to them that they hurt if I don't wear them. Go figure.

BEYONCÉ AND KELLY HAVE ALWAYS PERFORMED IN THE HIGHEST HEELS THEY COULD MANAGE. WHEN THEY WERE REALLY YOUNG IT WAS HARD FOR THEM TO DANCE IN HEELS. SO IN THE BEGINNING, THEY WORE PLATFORMS, WHICH WERE MUCH EASIER FOR THEM. AROUND AGE FIFTEEN OR SO THEY GRADUATED TO STILETTOS, AND ACTUALLY PRACTICED DANCING IN THEM. MICHELLE QUICKLY ADAPTED TO WEARING HEELS WHEN SHE JOINED THE GROUP. IT WAS TRICKY AT FIRST, BUT NOW IT'S SECOND NATURE. THESE DAYS, ALL OF THREE OF THEM COULD PROBABLY RUN A MARATHON WEARING HEELS IF THEY HAD TO.

VERY FEW PEOPLE ARE BORN WITH LEAN, MEAN LEGS, BUT WE CAN ALL LOOK LIKE WE HAVE THEM. THE TRICK IS FINDING THE RIGHT PAIR OF HEELS FOR YOUR NEEDS.

- If you have short legs, avoid platform-type chunky heels. It's okay to have a medium-sized platform in the front, but you want to make sure you have a thin heel in the back.
- If your legs are heavy, make sure the front of the shoe is substantial and has a low vamp. (The vamp is the upper front part of a boot or shoe.) Shoes that are too skimpy in the front or have a high vamp will make your feet look small compared to the rest of you.
- For skinny legs, light and airy-looking open-toed heels that show more skin are your best bet for making legs look proportionate. Mules are always flattering.
- For women with bowlegs, classic pumps with ornamentation near the arch look best. These shoes draw attention away from the inside of the leg. Over-the-knee pull-on boots are also good. Avoid calf-high boots.
- If you have big feet, try to stick to a high-arched heel with a semipointed toe or semisquared toe with no ornamentation.
- Small feet look proportional if you stick to a semipointed toe, a high vamp, and a heavy texture like brocade, snakeskin, or suede. Ankle-high boots or heels with ankle straps add the illusion of girth to narrow ankles.
- If you have wide ankles, shoes with a low vamp in dark matte colors give a slimming effect.

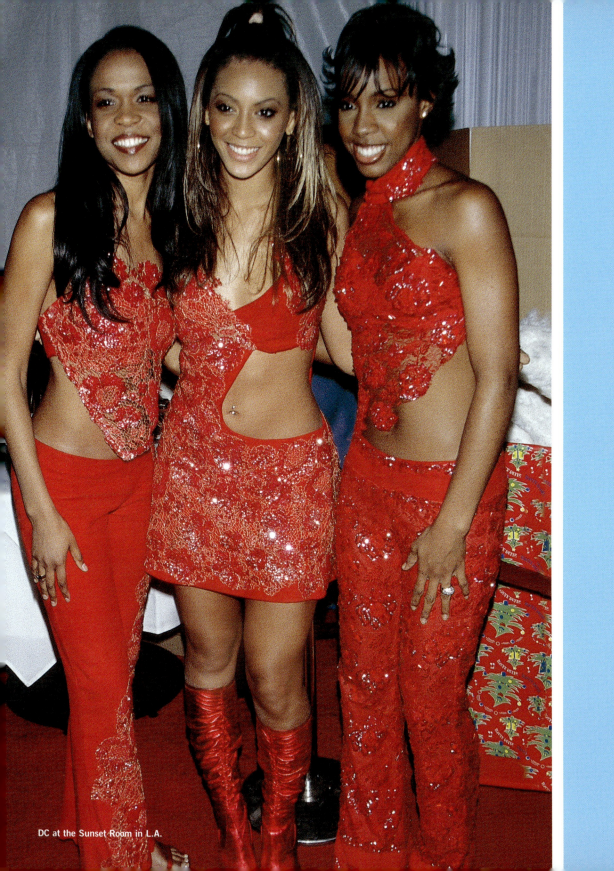

DC at the Sunset Room in L.A.

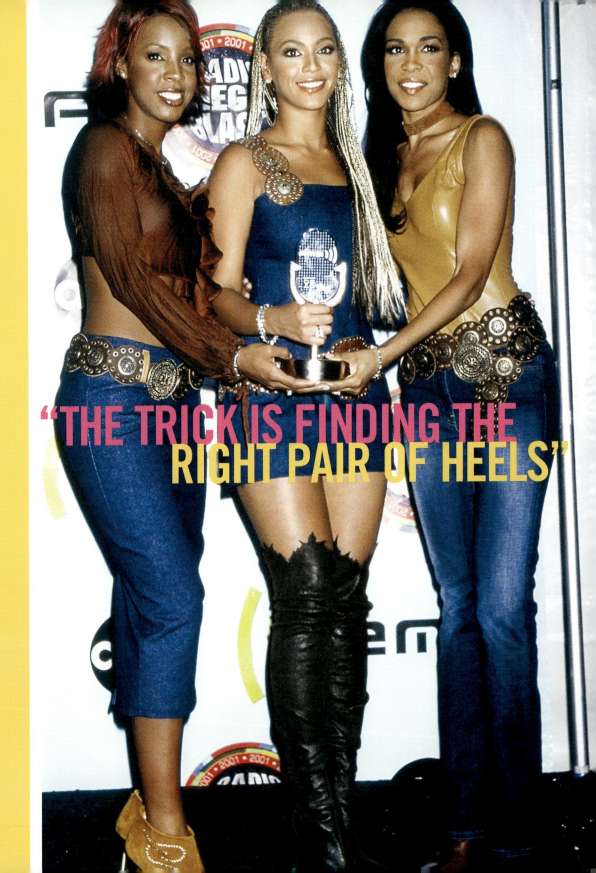

BOOTYLICIOUS SHOES

1. STILETTOS—THE HIGHER THE BETTER!
2. THIGH-HIGH BOOTS
3. COWBOY BOOTS WITH A POINTED TOE
4. STRAPPY SANDALS WITH A THIN HEEL

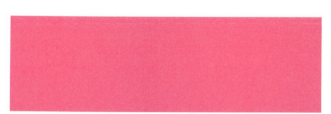

Funky boots on Beyoncé at the 2001 Radio Music Awards.

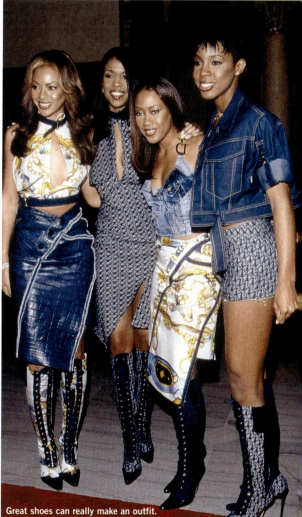

Great shoes can really make an outfit.

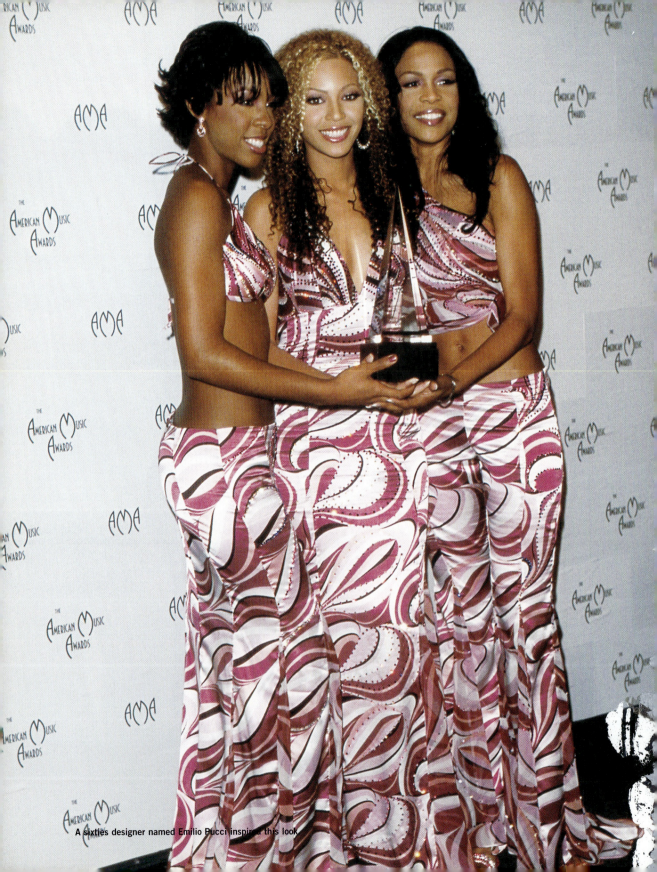

A sixties designer named Emilio Pucci inspired this look.

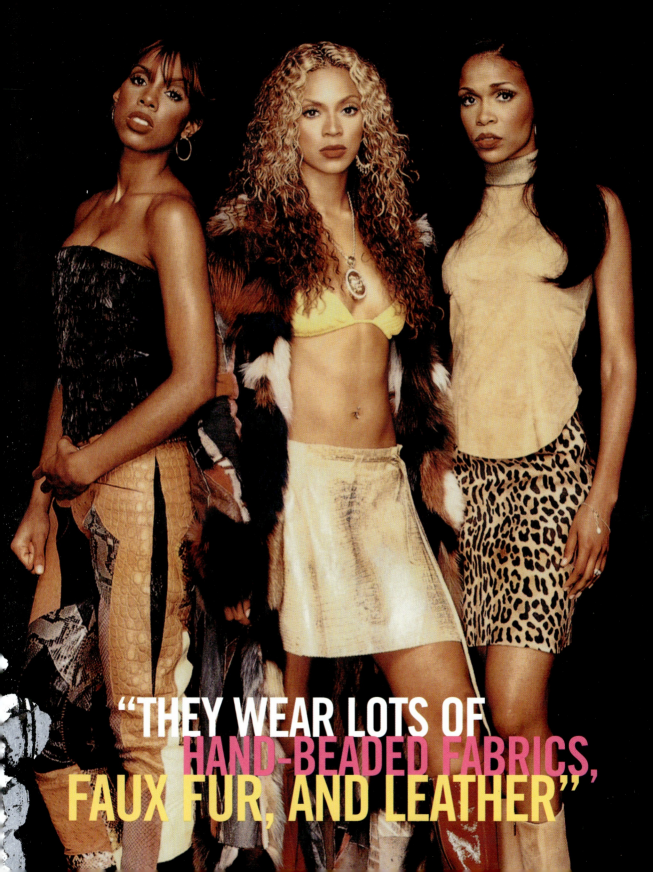

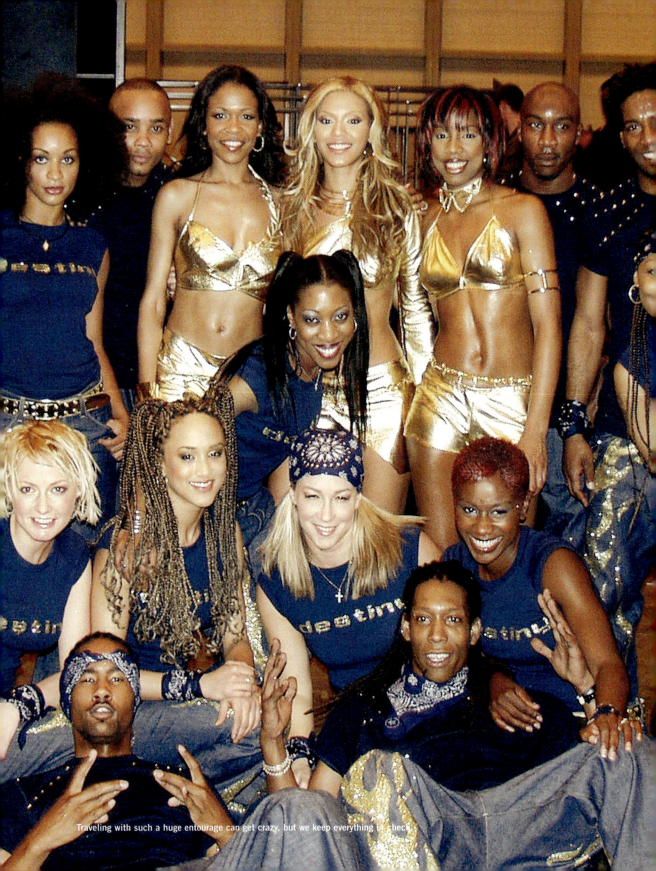

Traveling with such a huge entourage can get crazy, but we keep everything in check.

TAKING THE SHOW ON THE ROAD

THERE ARE CERTAIN THINGS THAT CAUSE PEOPLE TO TALK ABOUT RECORDING ARTISTS LIKE THEY'RE DOGS. ONE OF THEM IS THE SIZE OF THE ENTOURAGE, MEANING THE NUMBER OF PEOPLE WHO ACCOMPANY ARTISTS ON THE ROAD. AN ENTOURAGE IS NOT ALWAYS WHAT MOST PEOPLE THINK IT IS. YES, THERE ARE A FEW RECORDING ARTISTS WHO ROLL DEEP WITH YOGA INSTRUCTORS, FRIENDS, RELATIVES, PSYCHICS, LIVE ANIMALS, AND VARIOUS AND SUNDRY HANGERS-ON, IN ADDITION TO THE ESSENTIALS, LIKE THE BAND AND BACKUP SINGERS. HOWEVER, THE DC ENTOURAGE IS COMPOSED ONLY OF PEOPLE WE ACTUALLY NEED TO BE OUT ON THE ROAD WITH US TO MAKE THE SHOW HAPPEN. THAT IS MADE UP OF THE SECURITY; SOMETIMES A MAKEUP ARTIST; WARDROBE STYLIST (ME); MY WARDROBE ASSISTANT, TY; THE GIRLS' ASSISTANT, ANGIE; THE MUSICIANS; THE DANCERS; OUR PHOTOGRAPHER; AND A FEW TECHNICAL PEOPLE. THAT MAY SEEM LIKE A LOT OF PEOPLE, BUT IN ACTUALITY IT'S REALLY A THIN CREW, AND WE OPERATE LIKE A FAMILY.

"they improvised at the last minute by deconstructing their wardrobe"

One of the hazards that comes with this many people traveling is lost luggage. It's annoying when I'm traveling for recreation and a bag is lost. However, it's *devastating* when luggage containing one-of-a-kind costumes that DC is supposed to wear that same night goes missing. This has happened to us too many times to count, but the most heart-stopping time was when we flew to Washington, D.C., to perform at President George W. Bush's inauguration party. We arrived a few hours before the gig and, wouldn't you know it, the bag containing the DC costumes for the show was missing when we landed. As the hours ticked by, the airport had no luck locating the bag. So I hit the malls and shopping centers in the area to find outfits for them to wear. By the time I found a suitable replacement wardrobe, the girls had already been shuttled to the venue. Well, as you can imagine, since it was the presidential inauguration, security was tight. No one would let me into the facility to dress the girls. The cell phones wouldn't work inside, so there was no way to contact anyone to let them know I was outside trying to get in. None of the security believed that I, this harried-looking woman who was sweating and out of breath with shopping bags full of clothes was actually the stylist for Destiny's Child. Meanwhile, inside the venue, Beyoncé, Kelly, and Michelle realized that if they didn't do something, they'd be in trouble. So they improvised at the last minute by deconstructing their wardrobe. They cut up their T-shirts and pants and safety-pinned them back together. They went onstage and performed in those outfits and got rave reviews. They were featured in magazines all over the world and the response was overwhelmingly great. We lucked out, but that just goes to show it doesn't take a lot of money or time to put together a killer outfit.

So, now, to avoid lost-luggage woes like that one, I try to downsize the amount of personal luggage we bring on the road. It's hard enough to keep up with the trunks and bags that contain costumes, but when you factor in personal luggage, it's really a chore to keep up with everything. I learned how to pack efficiently in order to cut down on the amount of bags I had to keep track of.

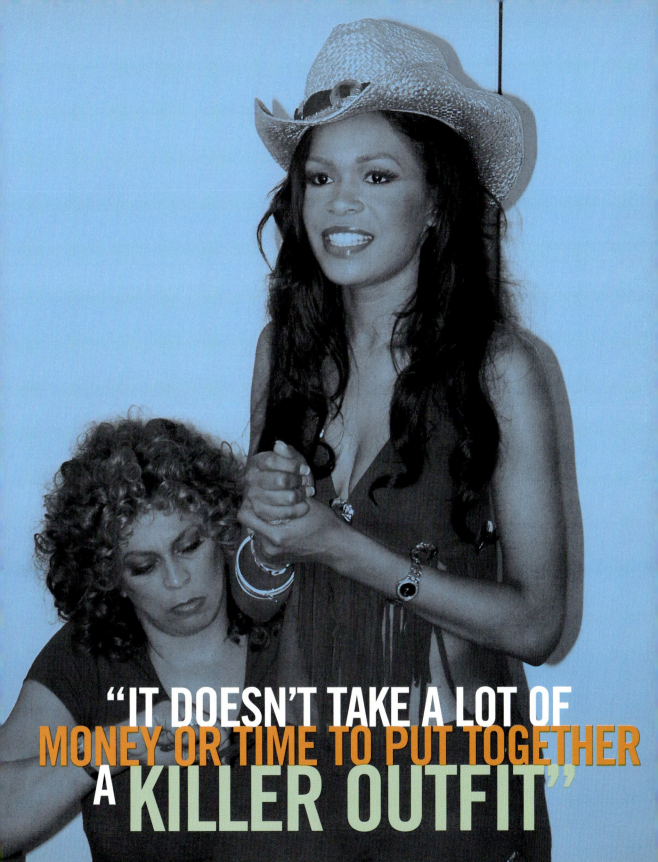

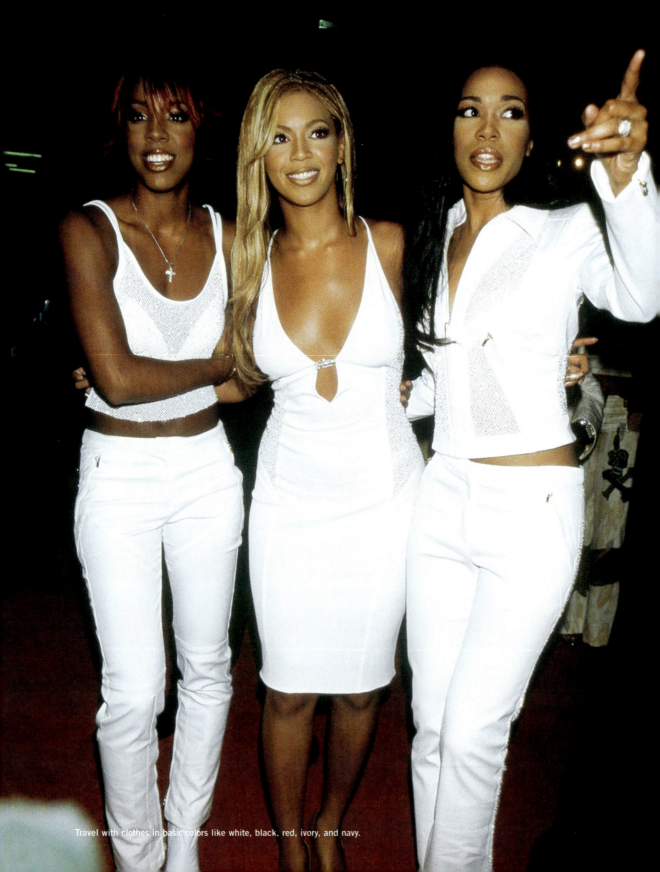
Travel with clothes in basic colors like white, black, red, ivory, and navy.

Wrinkle-free Packing

THE SECRET TO DC'S FASHION-ON-THE-GO IS ALL IN THE WAY I PACK. WHEN YOU'RE IN A HURRY AND NOT CAREFUL ABOUT CUTTING DOWN ON THE NUMBER OF BAGS YOU'RE CARRYING, YOU END UP STUFFING YOUR CLOTHES SO TIGHTLY INTO YOUR SUITCASES THAT THEY GET WRINKLED BEYOND RECOGNITION. I CAN'T TELL YOU HOW MANY TIMES WE'VE ARRIVED AT A HOTEL ROOM LATE AT NIGHT AND I'VE HAD TO STAY UP IRONING AND STEAMING DC COSTUMES SO THEY WOULD BE READY FIRST THING THE NEXT MORNING. IT WAS TIMES LIKE THOSE THAT MOTIVATED ME TO PACK THINGS CAREFULLY TO AVOID WRINKLING AS MUCH AS POSSIBLE. HERE ARE SOME HELPFUL TIPS:

- To save room, put your socks and underwear inside your shoes. Then slide the shoes into plastic bags to protect your clothing.
- Perfume bottles should also go inside your shoes. This protects the bottle and keeps your shoes from getting squished and losing their shape in your bag.
- Place heavy items at the very bottom or on the sides of your suitcase. This prevents them from falling down and wrinkling clothes when the suitcase is picked up.
- So you don't damage your luggage, high heels should be packed with the heel pointing toward the middle.
- Don't pack anything you wouldn't wear at home, because chances are you won't wear it while you're away either.
- Wrap necklaces on something round like a hair roller and then secure them with a rubber band. This prevents necklaces from getting all tangled up, which happens when you just throw them in a bag together.
- Travel with casual clothes in basic colors like black, white, ivory, red, and navy so you can easily mix and match, the exception being outfits for specific occasions you'll attend while traveling. The unofficial uniform for most of the DC crew when we're on the road seems to be blue jeans, a black turtleneck, and black boots. I don't know how it started, but all of us end up wearing this—probably because it's a no-brainer and it works. Easy outfits are key when we have to be up and ready to work at four o'clock in the morning after getting into bed at one.
- Always carry a small standard sewing kit. One that you can pick up at the drugstore for less than five dollars is fine. Be sure to bring small scissors and a lint brush as well.
- As soon as you arrive at your destination, unpack everything and hang any wrinkled clothes near the shower to steam away wrinkling while you bathe. If that doesn't cut it, most hotels will provide you with an iron and ironing board if you ask. So don't be afraid to request it.

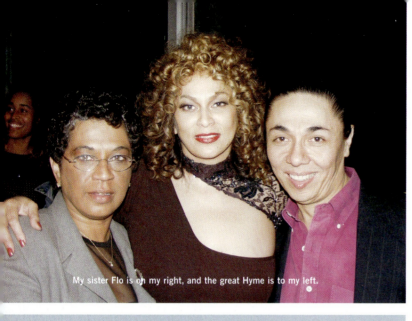
My sister Flo is on my right, and the great Hyme is to my left.

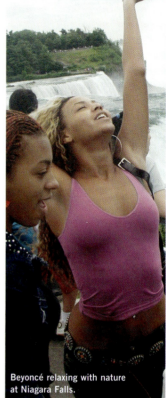
Beyoncé relaxing with nature at Niagara Falls.

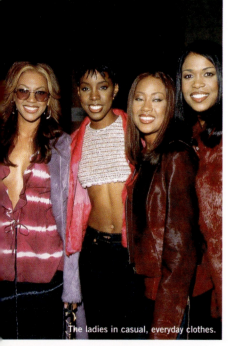
The ladies in casual, everyday clothes.

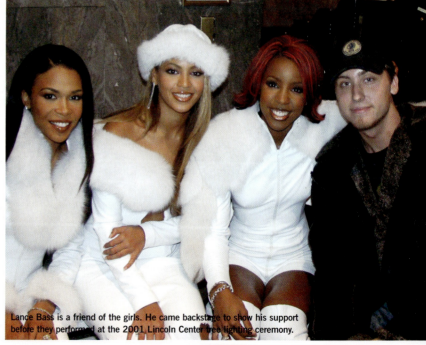
Lance Bass is a friend of the girls. He came backstage to show his support before they performed at the 2001 Lincoln Center tree lighting ceremony.

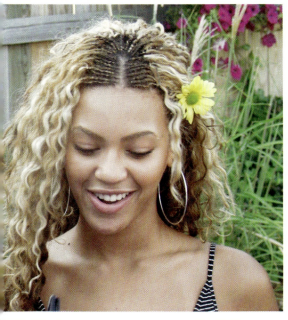

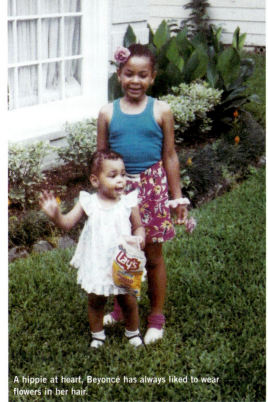

A hippie at heart, Beyoncé has always liked to wear flowers in her hair.

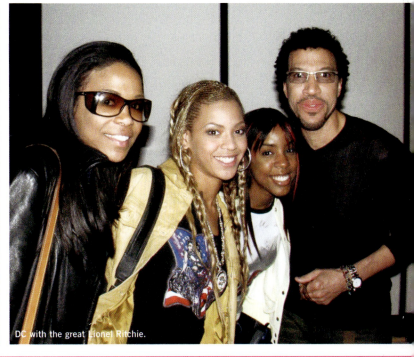

DC with the great Lionel Ritchie.

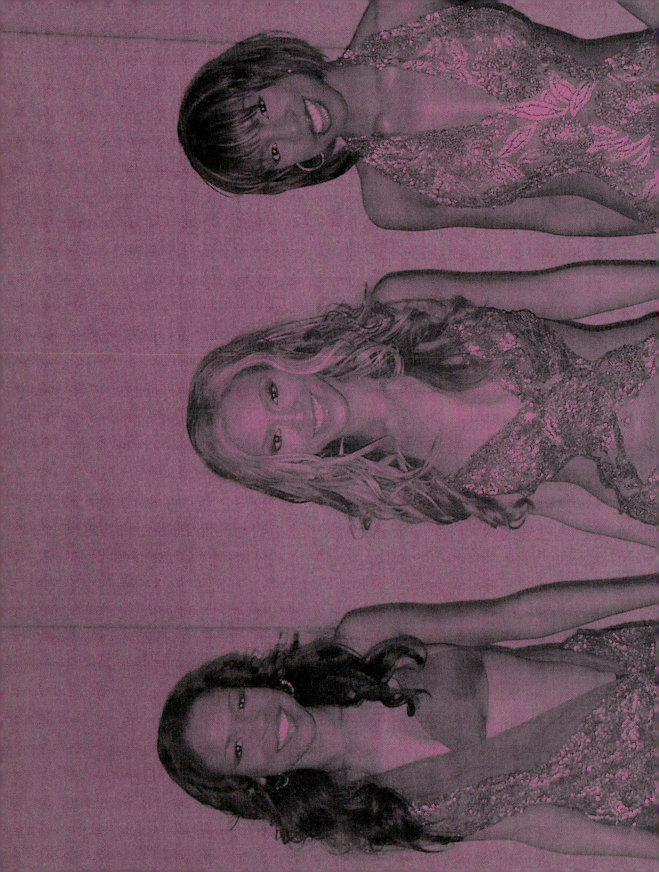

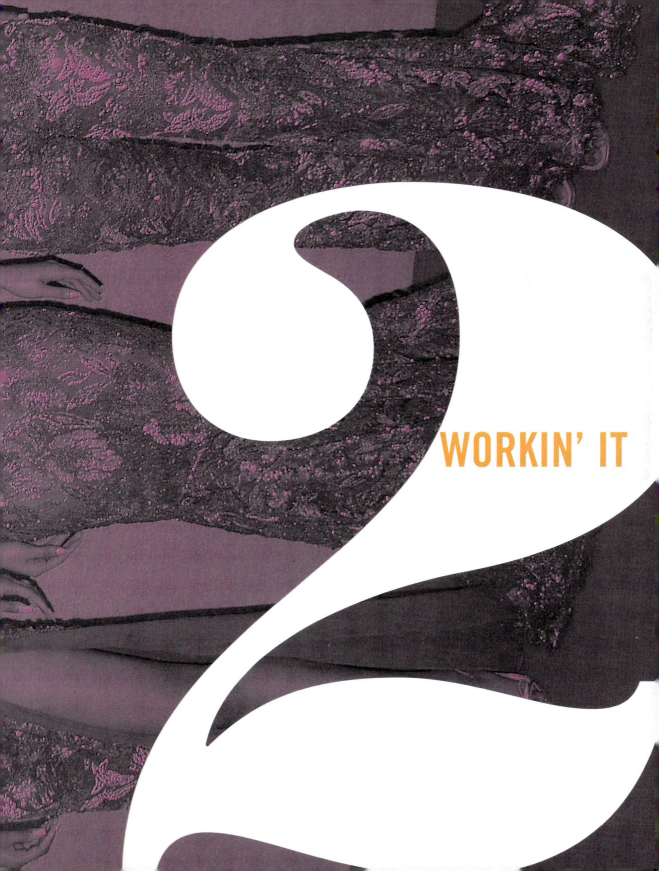

2 WORKIN' IT

THESE ARE GREAT TIMES FOR WOMEN TO FEEL GOOD ABOUT THEIR LOOKS. GONE ARE THE DAYS OF ONE STANDARD BEAUTY TYPE THAT EVERYBODY WAS TRYING TO LOOK LIKE. NOW, MORE THAN EVER, WOMEN OF ALL ETHNICITIES, SHAPES, AND SIZES REPRESENT THE MANY FACES OF BEAUTY IN THE MEDIA. ALL THE THINGS WE MAY HAVE BEEN TEASED ABOUT IN HIGH SCHOOL ARE IN FASHION NOW. THERE ARE MODELS OUT THERE WITH CROOKED NOSES, BOOTYLICIOUS BODIES, BIG FEET, HEAVY ANKLES, YOU NAME IT—IT'S OUT THERE. NOW THAT THE RULES OF BEAUTY HAVE CHANGED, ALL OF US CAN GIVE OURSELVES A BREAK AND BE OUR OWN INDIVIDUAL BEAUTIFUL SELVES.

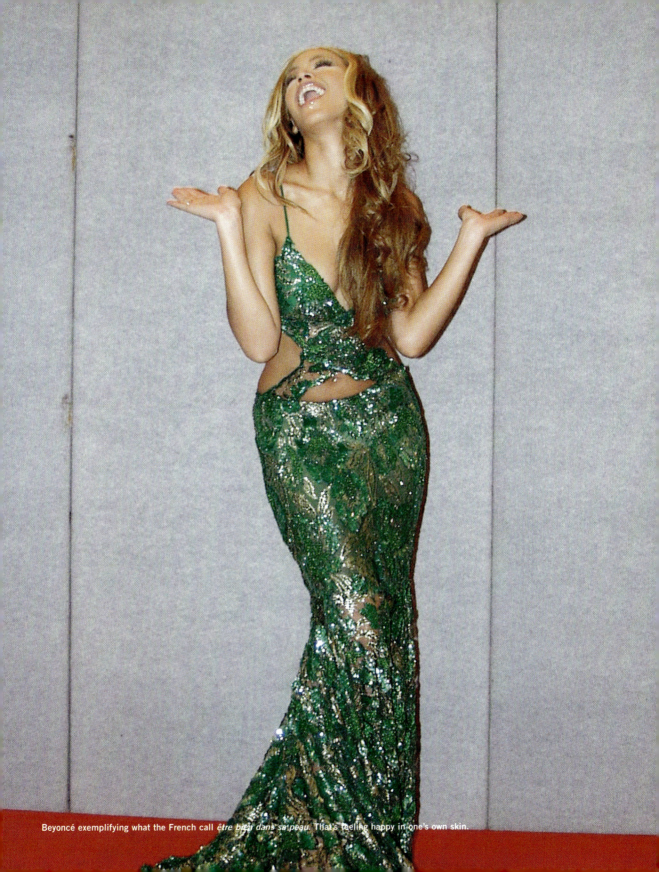

Beyoncé exemplifying what the French call *être bien dans sa peau*. That's feeling happy in one's own skin.

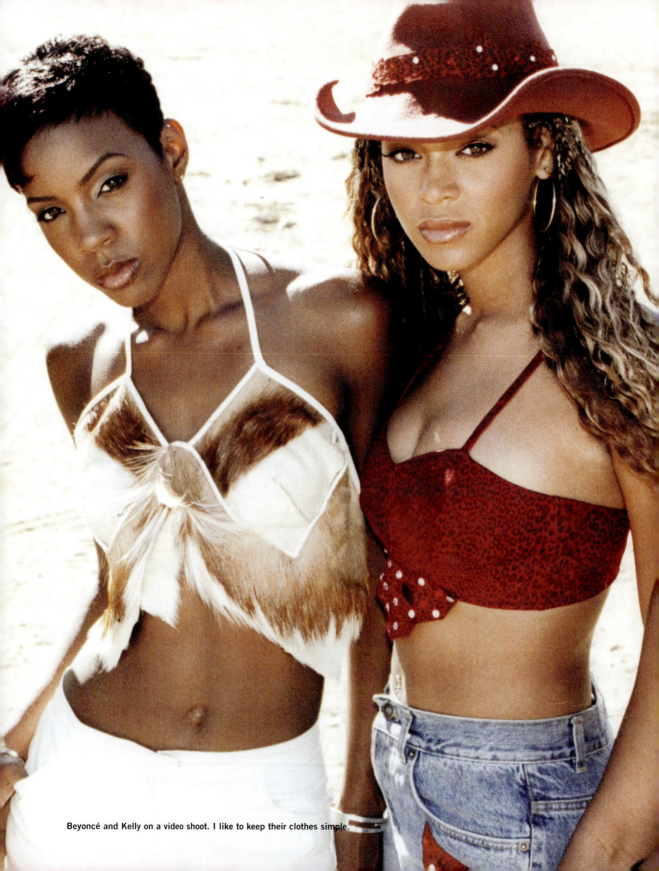

Beyoncé and Kelly on a video shoot. I like to keep their clothes simple.

SELECTING MORE "REAL-LOOKING" MODELS FOR AD CAMPAIGNS IS ONE WAY THAT DESIGNERS ARE MAKING HIGH FASHION AND BEAUTY MORE ACCESSIBLE TO THE AVERAGE PERSON. BEYONCÉ IS A PRIME EXAMPLE OF THIS. SHE WAS ASKED BY L'ORÉAL TO BE A SPOKESPERSON AND DO AN AD AS HERSELF, NOT AS A POP DIVA DECKED OUT IN HIGH-VOLTAGE HAIR AND MAKEUP. THE PHOTO L'ORÉAL USED IS HOW SHE NATURALLY LOOKS WITH VERY LITTLE MAKEUP AND AN EVERYDAY HAIRSTYLE IN A COLOR VERY CLOSE TO HER OWN. AT THE END OF THE DAY, WHEN SHE'S FINISHED PERFORMING, SHE'S JUST A NORMAL TWENTY-YEAR-OLD WOMAN AND THAT'S A SIDE HER AUDIENCE DOESN'T GET TO SEE IN DC VIDEOS. THAT'S WHY WE FELT THIS AD CAMPAIGN WAS SUCH A REFRESHING CHANGE.

Destiny's Child also tries to maintain a realistic image when it comes to their clothes. It would be a lot of fun for me to go to the most expensive boutiques in the world and select superexpensive, or "bling-bling," clothes for the girls to wear in their videos. I don't do this because most of the people watching the videos at home wouldn't be able to afford them. Chances are, if you see a pair of pants they are wearing in a video, you can hit the mall and find a similar pair. The thing about Beyoncé, Kelly, and Michelle is, even though they can afford to shop at high-priced boutiques, more often than not you'll find them at lower-priced department stores and at the mall. Since they wear affordable clothing at home, I feel it's important for them to wear similar clothes for public appearances as well.

The exceptions to this are huge events like award shows or big photo shoots. For those, I put the look together myself or I contact designers with whom I have a great working relationship, like Versace, and they invite me to their boutique or clothing showroom. There I "pull" clothes for the girls to wear for whatever the occasion might be. "Pulling" clothes is like borrowing books from a library. I pick out the outfits I like, and the store lends the clothes, shoes, and accessories to me. When the event or photo shoot is over, the garments are returned to the store in pristine condition. The reason this practice is so popular is that celebrities wear the borrowed clothes and are heavily photographed in them. Those pictures then show up in magazines all over the world. When people see a photo of a celebrity who has a style similar to theirs, they run to the store and say "I want the dress that so-and-so wore to the such-and-such awards." It ends up being a free advertisement for a designer.

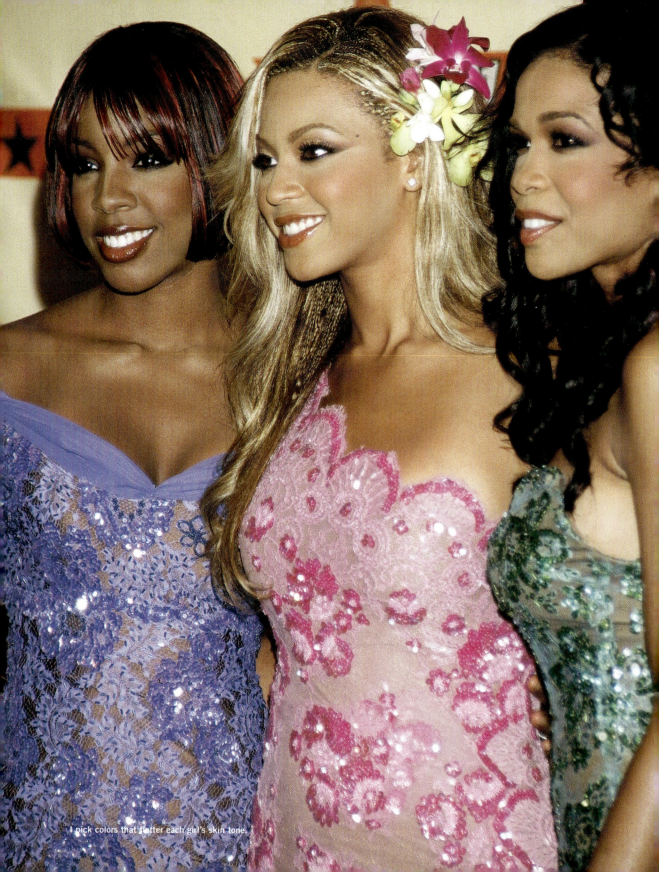

I pick colors that flatter each girl's skin tone.

STYLE vs. FASHION

IN THE FASHION WORLD, I'VE NOTICED THAT THE MINUTE "STYLE" BECOMES "FASHIONABLE"—MEANING EVERYONE'S WEARING IT—IT'S TIRED. I THINK HAVING STYLE IS MORE IMPORTANT THAN BEING IN FASHION, BECAUSE THE OUTCOME OF FASHION IS THAT EVENTUALLY EVERYONE ENDS UP LOOKING ALIKE. FASHION IS ABOUT THE CLOTHES. ANYBODY CAN GO TO THE STORE AND SEE WHAT'S "IN" THIS SEASON. WHAT MOST PEOPLE FIND CHALLENGING IS COMING UP WITH THEIR STYLE—SOMETHING THAT MAKES A STATEMENT ABOUT WHO THEY ARE OR THE IMAGE THEY'D LIKE TO PROJECT. HAVING REAL STYLE MEANS TAKING THE ESSENCE OF A LOOK YOU LIKE AND PERSONALIZING IT SO THAT IT LOOKS GOOD AND FEELS RIGHT ON YOU.

Most people are divided into two groups when it comes to style. There are the Constants, the people who pick a look and stick with it. Then there are the Chameleons, those who change their look every season or whenever they feel like it. A Constant simply updates her wardrobe with new pieces to keep things interesting and fresh while maintaining the essence of her look. For instance, Beyoncé and Solange favor clothing with an upscale hippie vibe. It's so much a part of their look that it's now become a part of their personalities. Their nonprofessional wardrobe consists of lots of jeans embroidered with butterflies and colorful stitching, crocheted and lace tops, and flowy dresses in earth tones. Their styles are so similar that they will often go shopping separately and come home with many of the exact same items. Michelle is also a Constant. She grew up having to wear skirts and dresses to church, so now she loves to wear pants whenever she can. She has the cutest collection of pantsuits, and whenever she sees a pair of pants she likes, she buys them. Pants are a part of who she is.

Then there are the Chameleons. These are people who change their look when it loses its "pop," when they feel like their look is "played out." Kelly is a Chameleon. She's always reconfiguring her own personal presentation. For her this can be as subtle as a new shade of lipstick or as drastic as a new shade of hair color. One day you'll see her in a man's suit and the next she'll be rockin' an ultrafeminine floor-length gown. It suits her personality, because one minute she can be singing a gospel hymn that will have you praising the Lord and the next she can break out into a hard-rock song and start slam-dancing. She has several sides to her, and she dresses to suit her mood.

Not everyone has the money to hire a stylist to shop for them. However, as quiet as it's kept, it's not a big, complicated thing to create a "look" that sets you apart as well as describes who you are. I taught myself to do it and so can you.

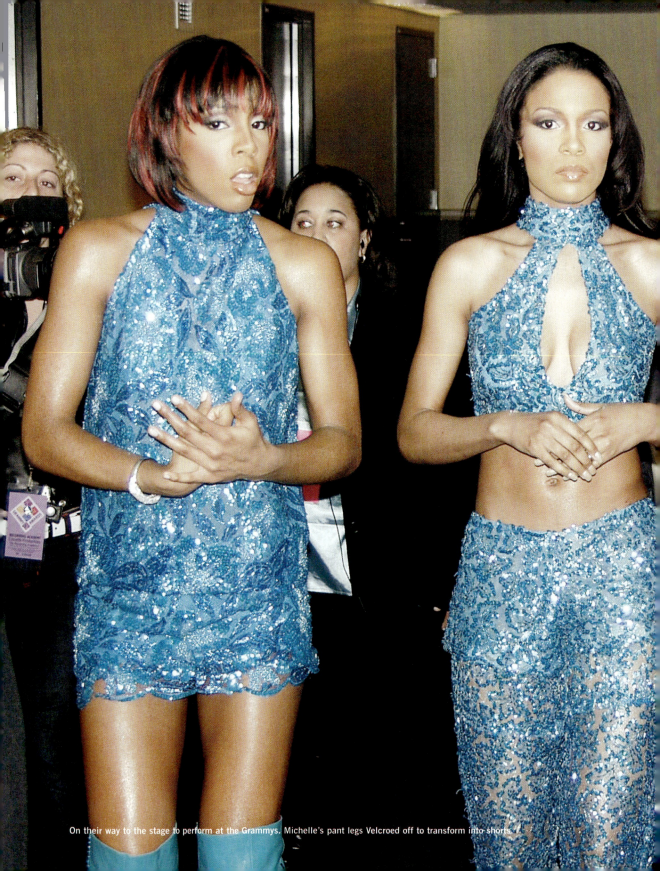

On their way to the stage to perform at the Grammys. Michelle's pant legs Velcroed off to transform into shorts.

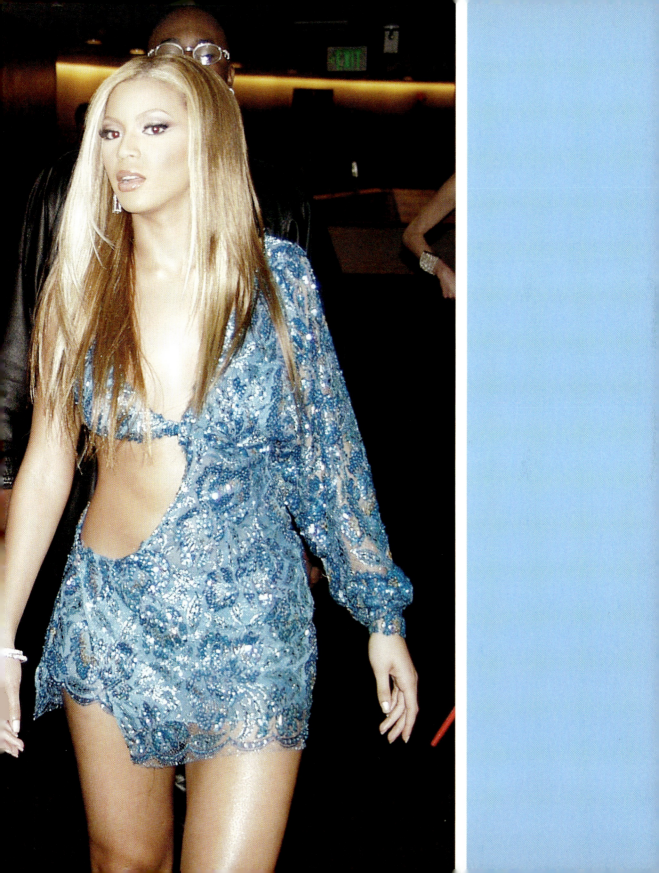

The Inspiration

I get letters from fans and people stop me on the street all the time to ask about the clothes that Beyoncé, Kelly, and Michelle wear onstage and in photos. The most popular question is, "How do you decide what they are going to wear?" Well, it's different every time, but I'll use the army camouflage look as an example because it's one of my favorites. I thought of putting the girls in camouflage because it fit the "survival" theme of the *Survivor* album. I try to make their outfits tie in to their songs.

The camouflage look worked so well that it became the rare exception to the rule that DC doesn't wear anything twice. They wore the outfits a lot while promoting the album and subsequently revived the camouflage trend. Pretty soon, I couldn't walk down the street without seeing someone wearing the camouflage look. Each time DC would wear their fatigue outfits, I'd do a little something different to them. For example, I applied rhinestones to the fatigues they wore for the Soul Train Awards and then again for the May 24, 2001, cover of *Rolling Stone*.

Sometimes I'll have a vision of what I want the group to wear and I'll spend a lot of time, effort, and money designing and customizing something only to not have it used—or if it is used, I'll get slammed for it. I was criticized by some people for the *Survivor* military fatigues. One general sent me a complaint letter because he was appalled that I'd cut up military uniforms for the girls to wear. But most heartbreaking is when an outfit can't be used. An example of this occurred in the most unlikely place of all—on the set of the children's TV show *Sesame Street*. The girls were so excited to be making an appearance on the show since it was a television institution that they enjoyed as kids. So I made special outfits for them to wear. I went to Kmart and bought a bunch of clothes that had *Sesame Street* characters sewn onto them and cut all the characters off. Then, using a hot-glue gun, I glued them onto some jeans. The jeans looked really nice with the colorful faces of Big Bird, Bert and Ernie, and Elmo on them. But when we arrived on the set, the head of the wardrobe department went ballistic. She said to me, "How would you like it if someone had taken your children's heads and sewn them onto clothes?" I couldn't understand her anger, but I meant no harm. I thought to myself, "My children's heads *are* on people's clothes." But, being the professionals the girls are, they took off the customized jeans and wore the plain jeans that they arrived in. It just goes to show you, no matter how old you get, there's always going to be someone who won't like your clothes.

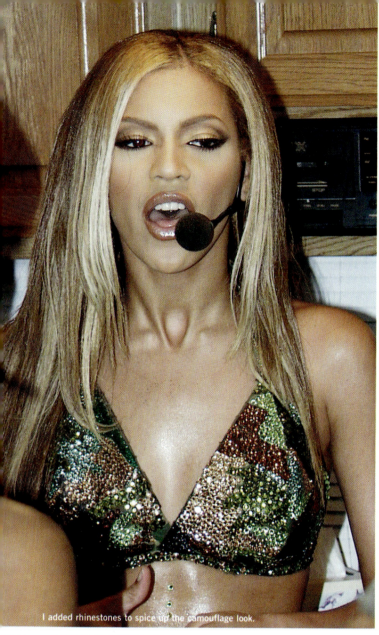

I added rhinestones to spice up the camouflage look.

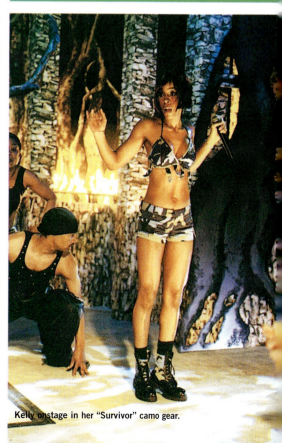

Kelly onstage in her "Survivor" camo gear.

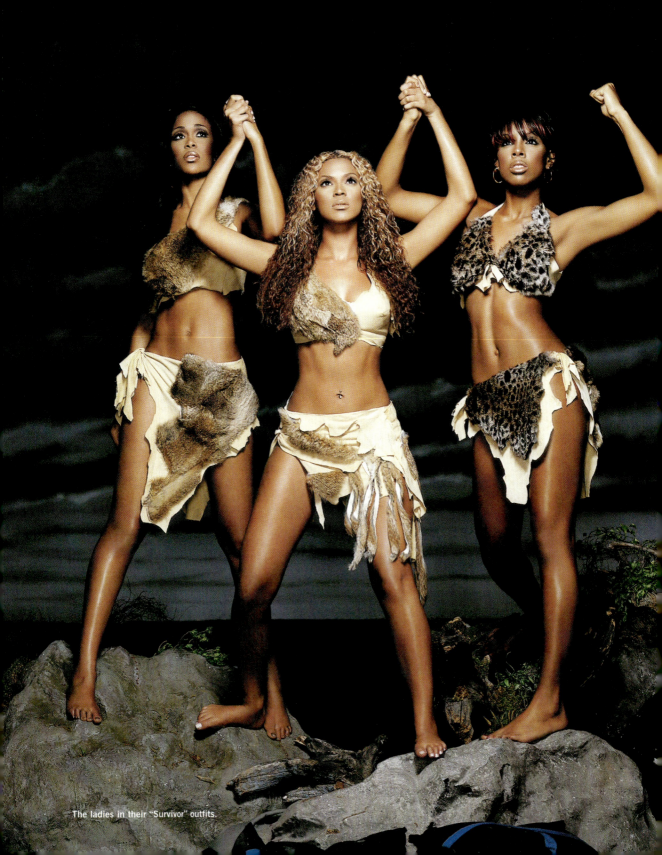
The ladies in their "Survivor" outfits.

Coming up with new ideas isn't always easy. Sometimes when I have a dress to make I don't have any ideas of what I want the girls to wear, so I go to the fabric store and hang out. As I look at all the materials, ideas come into my head and I start envisioning different outfits.

For last year's MTV Video Music Awards, I envisioned the ladies wearing suede. So I sent a coral color swatch to the fabric manufacturer. The following day suede material in the shade I asked for arrived, and I sat down and made a rough sketch of the outfits for Hyme, who sews most of DC's outfits for me. As I was sketching, I decided I wanted to incorporate turquoise into the outfits, so I purchased some turquoise jewelry. Once the outfits were completed, I spray-painted and customized matching shoes.

The things I use most often for inspiration are magazines, old movies, TV shows, and other people. Magazines are an invaluable tool to track a variety of new looks. Just pick up your favorite entertainment or fashion magazine and start browsing. You can rip out pictures and keep them in a folder to refer back to. You may get hooked and start keeping notebooks full of clippings with subdividers for shoes, hats, and belts. Just don't get too carried away or you'll start to become a pack rat. I keep a notebook handy to jot down ideas, which works best for me since I'm always on the go. When you start to really pay attention, you'll notice that you have a preference for certain clothes or celebrities' styles that "speak" to you. We are always browsing through magazines while at the airport or on the plane. I take notes on clothes I think will look good on the girls, and then I work their personal style into it. I look at all types of magazines for inspiration, but I find international fashion magazines are the most avant-garde so they spark my creativity.

Old movies are great for analyzing fashion because you can rent a bunch of movies by theme, time period, or with the actress whose look you most like. Then you can figure out new and inventive ways to re-create those looks. We have a collection of Marilyn Monroe movies, such as *Some Like It Hot* and *How to Marry a Millionaire*. The girls in those movies wore some of the baddest dresses you've ever seen. I've designed some DC gowns with that in mind. The knee-length white lace dresses the ladies wore on *Oprah* when they were promoting their album *8 Days of Christmas* were inspired by an old black-and-white movie I caught one night while channel surfing. The fur ensembles Beyoncé, Kelly, and Michelle wore in the "Survivor" video were inspired by the movie *One Million Years B.C.* starring Raquel Welch. I even styled Beyoncé's hair to look exactly like Raquel Welch's hair in the famous movie poster.

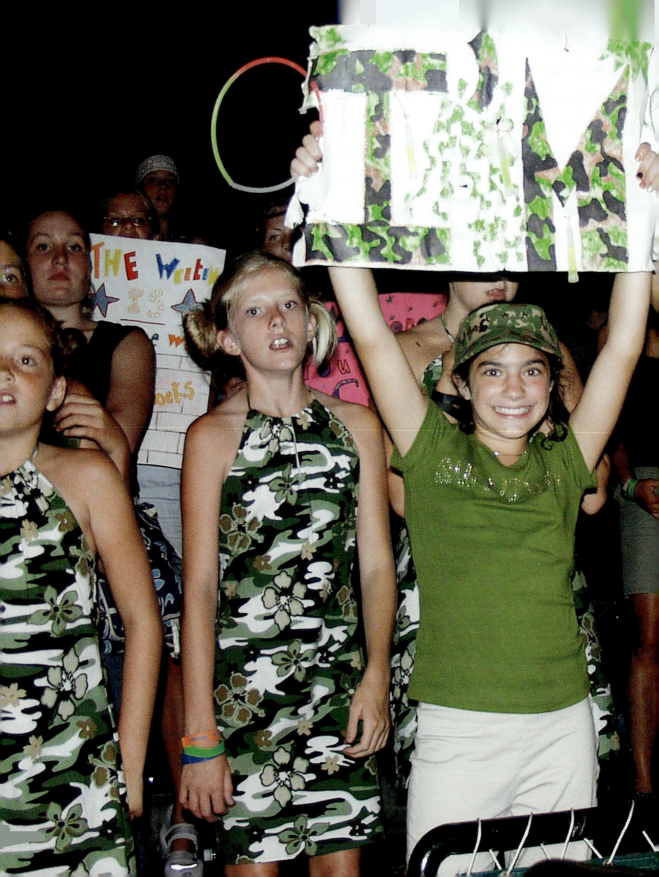

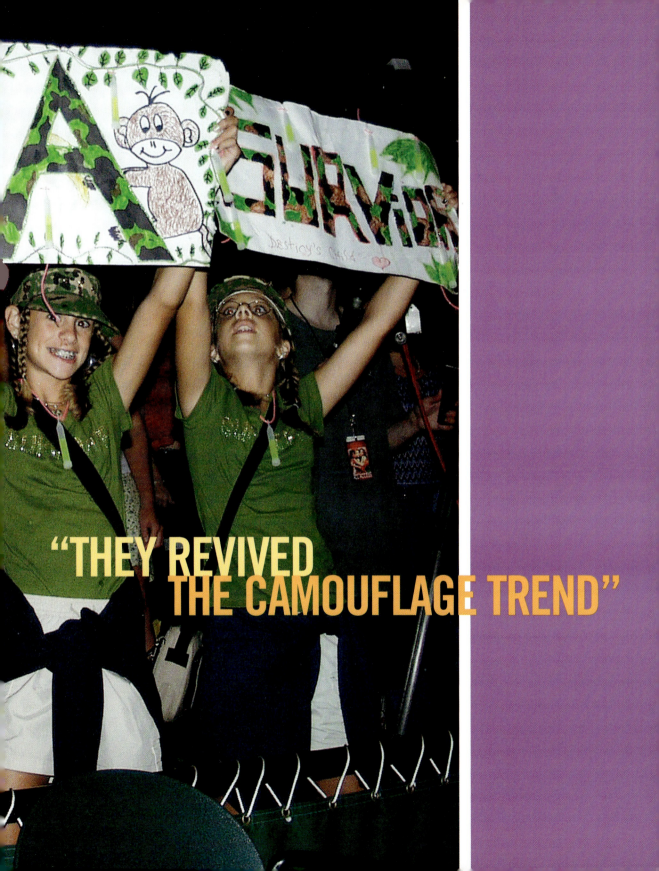

"THEY REVIVED THE CAMOUFLAGE TREND"

"i look at all types of magazines for inspiration"

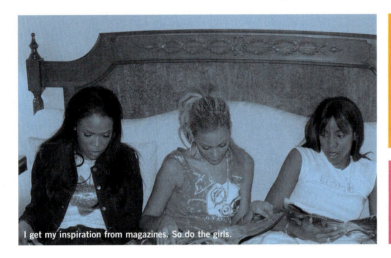

I get my inspiration from magazines. So do the girls.

Television is another brilliant source for wardrobe inspiration. Sometimes on late-night cable I catch old clips of Motown groups performing on *The Ed Sullivan Show* or old *Sonny and Cher Show* episodes. Reruns are very important to me because I draw a lot of inspiration from that time in my life. It was from watching Cher in her sparkly, eye-catching outfits that my concept of how a star should dress was formed. From the beginning, I've tried to maintain a glitzy and glamorous look for DC, like the old Motown look when all the women wore beautiful gowns and had flawless hair and makeup. When you're a star, you should look like a star. Besides, all the rhinestones and iridescent colors are fun.

People watching is another great source fashion ideas. Because DC travels so much, we are exposed to hundreds of different styles every time we go to a new place. DC has very fashionable fans. If the girls or I see a fan rocking an accessory or wearing something we think is interesting, I might incorporate it into a look for the group. Style is everywhere. If you keep your eyes open, you'll be constantly inspired.

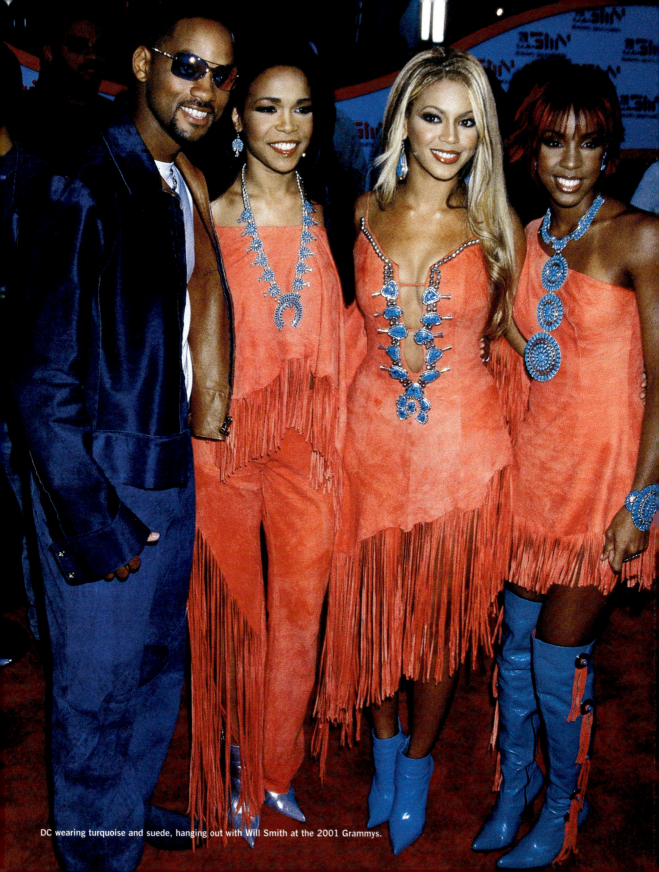

DC wearing turquoise and suede, hanging out with Will Smith at the 2001 Grammys.

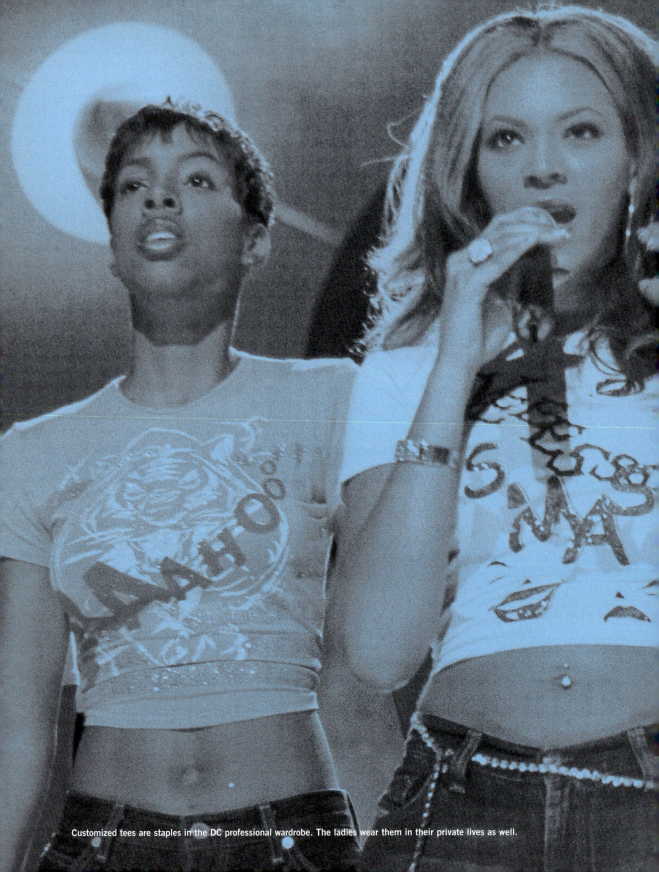
Customized tees are staples in the DC professional wardrobe. The ladies wear them in their private lives as well.

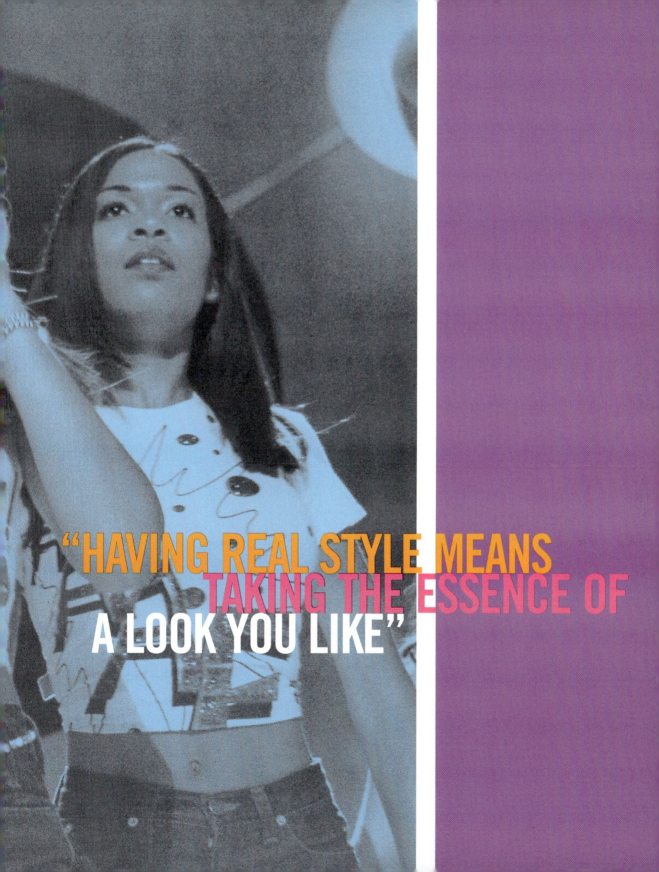

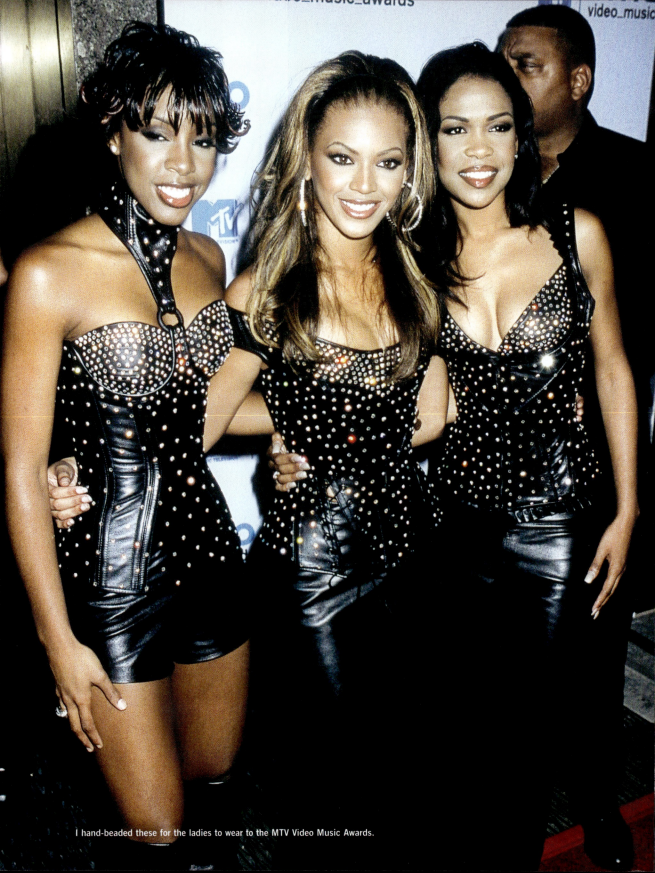

I hand-beaded these for the ladies to wear to the MTV Video Music Awards.

CUSTOMIZING YOUR STYLE

WHEN DESTINY'S CHILD WAS PROMOTING THEIR SELF-TITLED DEBUT ALBUM ON COLUMBIA, THEY WERE PERFORMING AND BEING INTERVIEWED ALMOST EVERY DAY. MATHEW HAD ALWAYS STRESSED THAT ONE ELEMENT OF DC'S LOOK SHOULD BE THAT THEY NEVER WEAR THE SAME THING TWICE. NOW THAT DC IS ONE OF THE TOP-SELLING GROUPS IN THE WORLD, WE'RE GIVEN A BUDGET TO MAKE THIS HAPPEN. THE GIRLS GO THROUGH SO MANY OUTFITS THAT THERE'S AN ENTIRE ROOM AT MY HUSBAND'S RECORD LABEL, MUSIC WORLD, THAT'S FULL OF THEIR OLD ONES. MANY OF THE OUTFITS WE DONATE TO CHARITY, AND ONE OF OUR FAVORITES IS ROSIE O'DONNELL'S EBAY AUCTION. SOMETIMES I GIVE OUTFITS AWAY TO FRIENDS, BUT WE KEEP MOST OF THE SHOES. I HAVE STACKS AND STACKS OF THEM LINING THE SHELVES OF MY BEDROOM'S WALK-IN CLOSET, BUT IT WASN'T ALWAYS SO.

> "customizing is one of the activities we bond over"

Back in the early days of Destiny's Child, every time the girls wore an outfit, it hurt me to have to retire it. Record companies don't usually spend a lot of money on new artists when they are first starting. In DC's case, Columbia wasn't really thrilled with the fact that I was making their outfits, so the record company didn't really give me much of a budget to work with. Columbia figured if "Mom" was making the outfits, they couldn't cost much. Basically I got a budget that would have been modest even if there had been only one girl in the group, but at the time the lineup consisted of four girls. Let me tell you, stretching that budget to accommodate all of them was sometimes rough. That's when customizing saved the day. I could go to the mall or a discount store and pick out four really inexpensive pairs of jeans and make them look like one-of-a-kind designer originals by adding little embellishments made of fabric patches or inexpensive lace appliqués. Then I would buy some inexpensive material and sew different-shaped tops for each of the girls to wear.

Customizing is one of the activities we bond over. Kelly has customized shirts for Beyoncé, and Beyoncé has customized jeans for both Kelly and Michelle. Whenever they have free time, which is almost never these days, they can be found making something while knee-deep in fabric, glitter, and glue. Every one of the ladies is artistic and, depending on her mood, her creativity will come out in different ways.

The home base for most of our rhinestone and glitter projects is the island in the middle of my kitchen. Of all the girls, Kelly's the most frequent customizer. She'll get on glittering kicks with shirts. She's really creative. She'll go through periods where she customizes shirt after shirt after shirt. One of Beyoncé's favorite shirts is one that Kelly customized for her with David Bowie's face on it. Kelly glittered it by hand. Beyoncé wanted him to have a gold tooth, so Kelly did it. She's good, because she is really patient and takes her time.

An example of how a little fabric can go a long way.

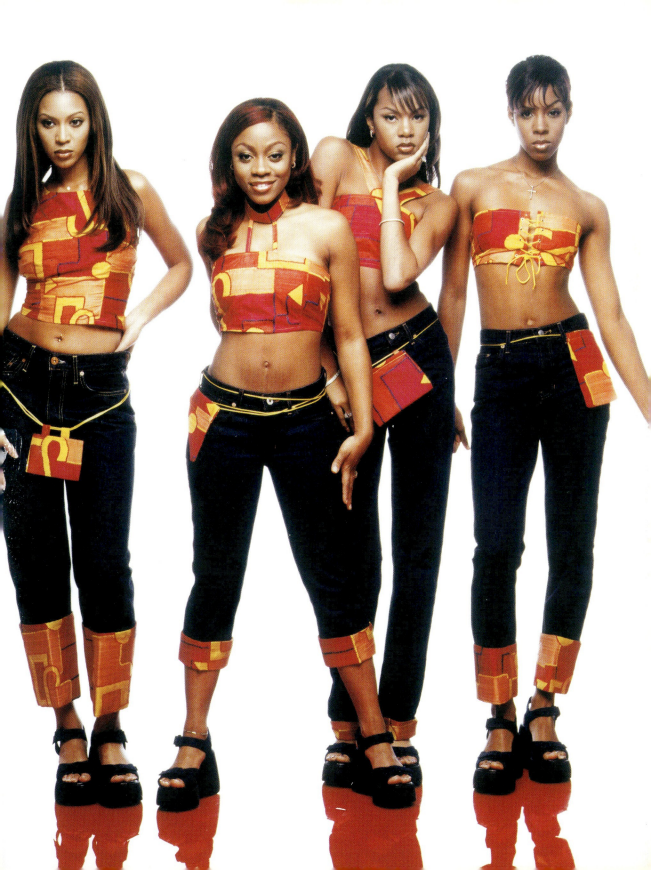

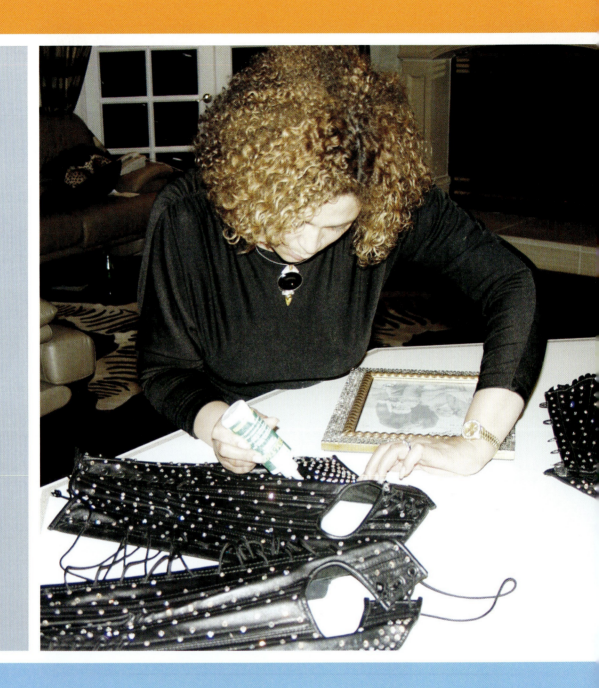

Anyone can customize. Even if you think you're not creative, you should try it, because you'll probably surprise yourself. I remember one night a few years ago, my niece Angie saw me running around trying to finish up the girls' costumes for a show the following day. She made the mistake of asking me if there was anything she could do to help. Well, she'd never customized a thing before, but faster than you could say "boo" I had her out in the garage spray-painting boots gold and then adding rhinestones. She didn't know what to do with herself when I first gave her the instructions. She was afraid she would mess up the boots because she'd never done anything like that before. I told her to cover the shoes in paint, except for the heel. Then add rhinestones to the heel. She panicked and said, "I don't know how to do this, Aunt Tina." I told her to make a design with the different color rhinestones and keep adding to it until the heel was covered. She started adding the little rhinestones hesitantly at first, but by the time she was finished with the first shoe, she was into it and excited to start on the others. She never considered herself an artist, but the pride she felt when creating customized shoes was inspiring. Now whenever there's customizing to be done, Angie's the first one to volunteer. Pretty much anyone who's around me and has a free hand ends up customizing at some point. I've recruited many many innocent friends and people from the record company, like Michelle Welsh and Yvette Noel-Schure, who have come to my home and ended up in front of a box full of rhinestones creating something.

The great thing about customizing is that your creations can be as simple or as intricate as your skill level allows. All you need is a tube of fabric glue—and there are plenty on the market. The most popular for rhinestoning are Beacon's Gem-Tac and, my personal favorite, Aleene's Jewel-It. Then go to the local craft store and pick up some rhinestones in colors you like or that match the T-shirt or whatever it is you want to customize. Once you have your supplies and your T-shirt is laid out in front of you, start with something easy, like putting a star on the front of the shirt. You can draw the star with a fabric pen or Magic Marker to make a guide for yourself. Then glue the rhinestones over what you traced. It's that simple. If you want, you can leave it that way or you can keep going and fill in the middle of the star with more rhinestones.

"anyone can customize"

Me, hand-beading the costumes that DC wore for the MTV Video Music Awards. I also made a picture frame.
Rhinestones are so versatile—you can use them on almost anything.

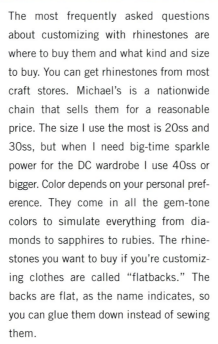

The most frequently asked questions about customizing with rhinestones are where to buy them and what kind and size to buy. You can get rhinestones from most craft stores. Michael's is a nationwide chain that sells them for a reasonable price. The size I use the most is 20ss and 30ss, but when I need big-time sparkle power for the DC wardrobe I use 40ss or bigger. Color depends on your personal preference. They come in all the gem-tone colors to simulate everything from diamonds to sapphires to rubies. The rhinestones you want to buy if you're customizing clothes are called "flatbacks." The backs are flat, as the name indicates, so you can glue them down instead of sewing them.

As with real jewels, there are several levels of quality in rhinestones. Swarovski Austrian crystal rhinestones are made from leaded crystal, and they are the standard by which all other rhinestones are measured. They have a superior cut, which means they have extra "bling-bling" appeal. Basically, they are expensive. You get about fifty for nine or ten dollars, so to stud an outfit or a pair of shoes can cost a fortune. However, they are great if you want to make your own jewelry or hair accessories because you don't need that many. The second best in quality are crystal rhinestones that are manufactured in the Czech Republic. The other option is good old acrylic rhinestones. They may not have the international pedigree of the other two, but they get the job done and don't cost an arm and a leg. You can get a bag of a hundred or so for around seven or eight dollars. I prefer Swarovski for intense sparkle power. These days we have a healthy wardrobe budget to afford them. When shopping for crystals, it pays to shop for the best price.

You'll be amazed at how addictive customizing can be. It starts with a T-shirt, and then you find yourself adding some rhinestones to a purse or the straps on a pair of sandals. Next thing you know, you're dyeing a concert T-shirt and adding some glitter. Pretty soon, half your wardrobe's customized. It's a fun hobby that everyone in the family can enjoy. My youngest daughter, Solange, is a recording artist now, but when she was younger, she used to be my little helper when it came time to customize. She's very creative. She takes jeans and creates designs on them using bleach. She fringes them and does all kinds of things I would have never thought of. She has helped me come up with some of the customized looks I've designed for DC.

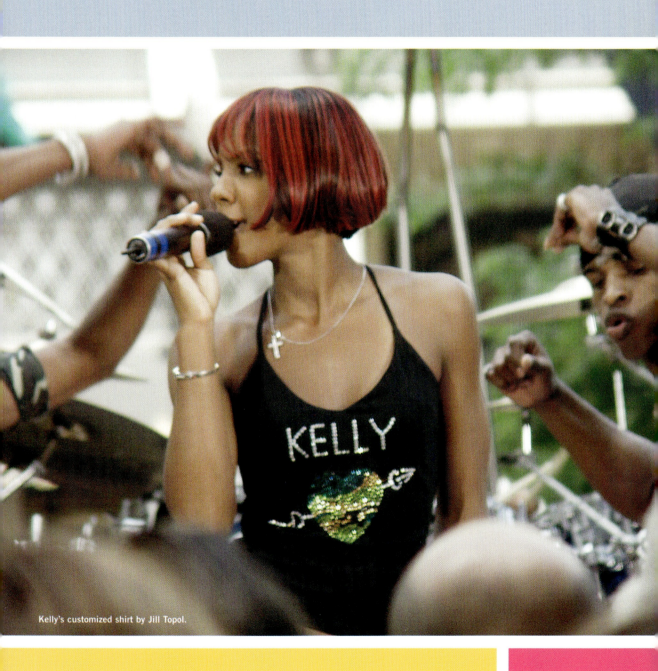
Kelly's customized shirt by Jill Topol.

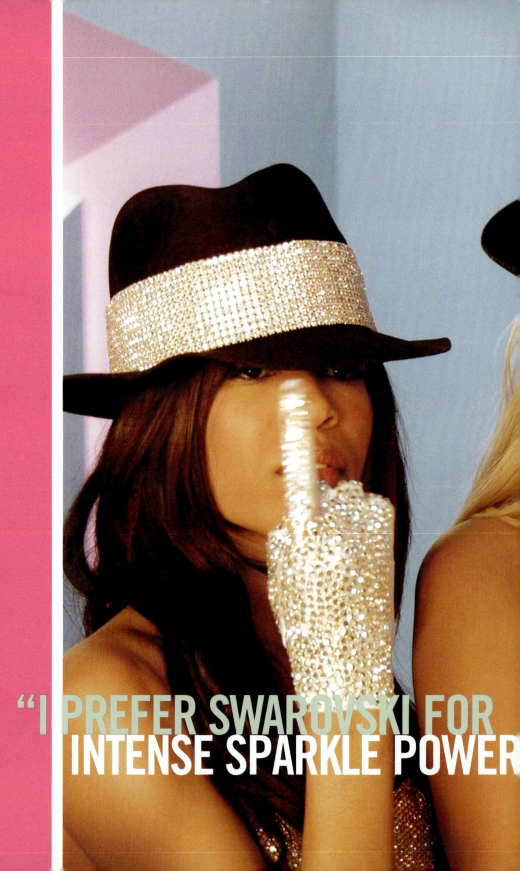

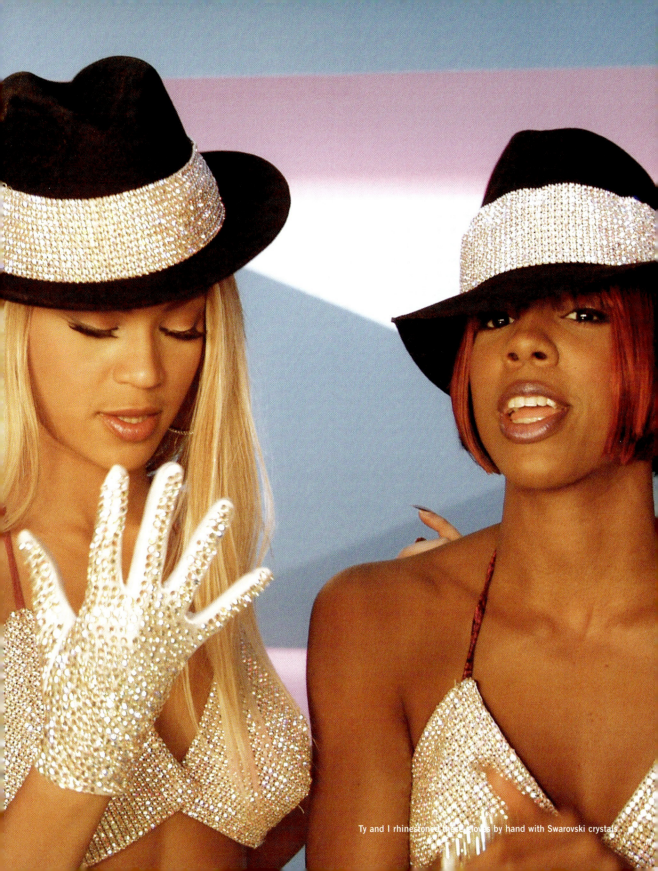

Ty and I rhinestoned these gloves by hand with Swarovski crystals.

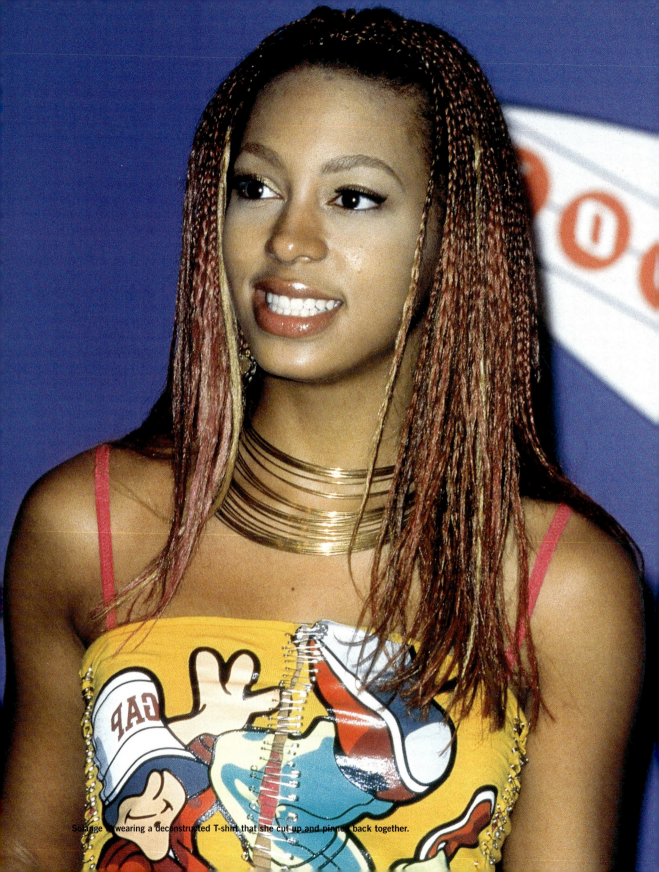

Solange is wearing a deconstructed T-shirt that she cut up and pinned back together.

Deconstruction

Another popular customizing technique is deconstruction. Remember the inauguration outfits I told you about? When Beyoncé, Kelly, and Michelle cut up their T-shirts and pinned them back together, they were deconstructing them. Here's how you can do it:

- Get a box of safety pins and a plain white crew-neck T-shirt. I look for the least expensive ones in the men's department of discount stores like Target or Wal-Mart.

- Cut the bottom off the T-shirt, just above the hem.

- Then fray the collar with your scissors by cutting it any way that you like.

- Cut slits in the T-shirt any way that feels good to you. (It's strangely therapeutic.)

- Then take the safety pins and secure them onto the slits like you're trying to close them up.

If you want, you can customize the shirt further by dyeing or gluing on rhinestones. You can deconstruct anything. Add new life to old T-shirts by deconstructing them or jazz up a pair of jeans. Go to the Salvation Army and buy a pair of worn jeans. They are great to use when you practice deconstructing because they don't cost much and if you mess up, it's not an expensive mistake because they are still good for patchworking.

The financial savings you get from customizing are unequaled. We've all had those days when you're ready to overhaul your whole wardrobe but your pocketbook just can't manage it. Customizing can help you transform your wardrobe without dropping a lot of dough.

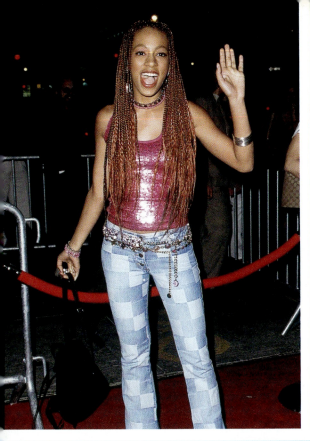
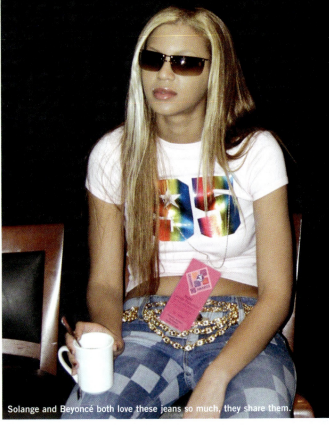
Solange and Beyoncé both love these jeans so much, they share them.

DECONSTRUCTED JEANS

BEYONCÉ HAS ALWAYS LOVED TO CUT UP JEANS. SHE WAS DECONSTRUCTING JEANS BEFORE THERE WAS A NAME FOR IT. HERE'S AN EASY METHOD FOR DECONSTRUCTING A PAIR OF JEANS.

1. CUT OFF ONE OF THE BACK POCKETS, BEING CAREFUL NOT TO CUT THROUGH THE BUTT OF THE JEANS.

2. OPEN THE SEAMS OF THE HEM AT THE BOTTOM OF THE LEGS WITH A SEAM RIPPER. (YOU CAN GET ONE FROM THE FABRIC STORE.)

3. UNFOLD THE EXTRA FABRIC THAT YOU'LL FIND ONCE THE HEMS ARE OPEN. YOU'LL SEE THAT YOU HAVE A FRAYED "DESCONTRUCTED" LOOK. AFTER YOU WASH THE JEANS THEY'LL HAVE AN EVEN MORE INTENSE DECONSTRUCTED LOOK.

4. THEN CUSTOMIZE THEM BY USING APPLIQUES OR A BEDAZZLER.

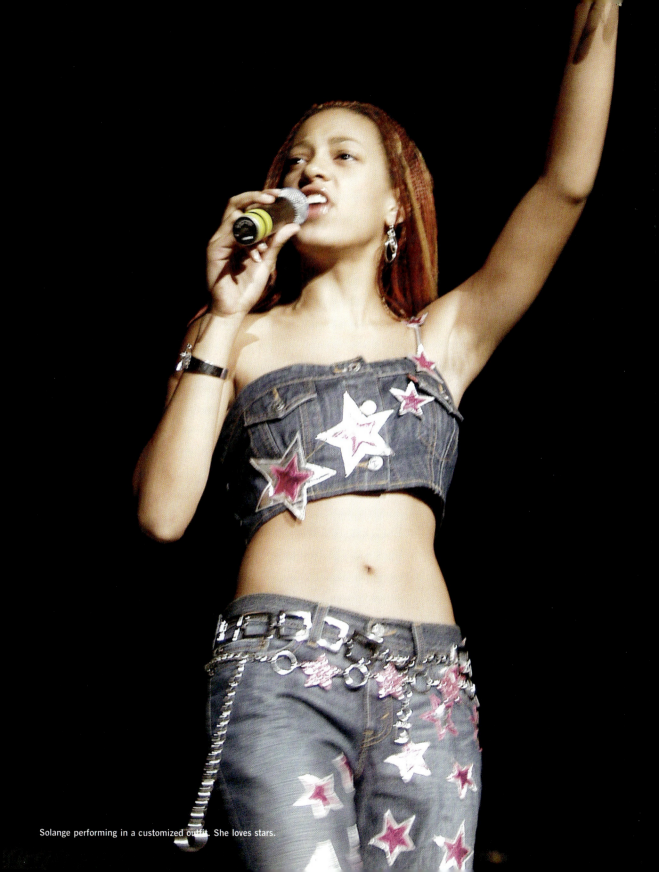
Solange performing in a customized outfit. She loves stars.

CUSTOMIZING KIT

HERE ARE SOME OF THE SUPPLIES I TAKE WITH ME ON THE ROAD IN MY CUSTOMIZING KIT. YOU MAY NOT NEED ALL THESE THINGS. YOU CAN PURCHASE THEM AS THE NEED ARISES.

- *A box of different colored rhinestones.* Use them to dress up shoes, shirts, and jeans. I've taken an inexpensive pair of shoes and rhinestoned them to create an expensive and fabulous look.
- *Beads.* They can be strung together to make necklaces and bracelets, or used to trim pants or shirt cuffs.
- *Patches.* I use patches on the ladies' jeans all the time. I keep all kinds, from Girl Scout patches to motorcycle patches. I never know how I'll use them.
- *Buttons.* Always save buttons—you never know when you'll need one. Interesting ones can be used to dress up a boring top or jacket.
- *Eyelet hole puncher.* These are great for shirts, boots, pants—you name it. One of my favorite looks is to take a pair of jeans and use the eyelet hole puncher to punch holes on the sides. I then thread them up using ribbons or scarves.

Kids loved this deconstructed T-shirt, and so did the paparazzi.

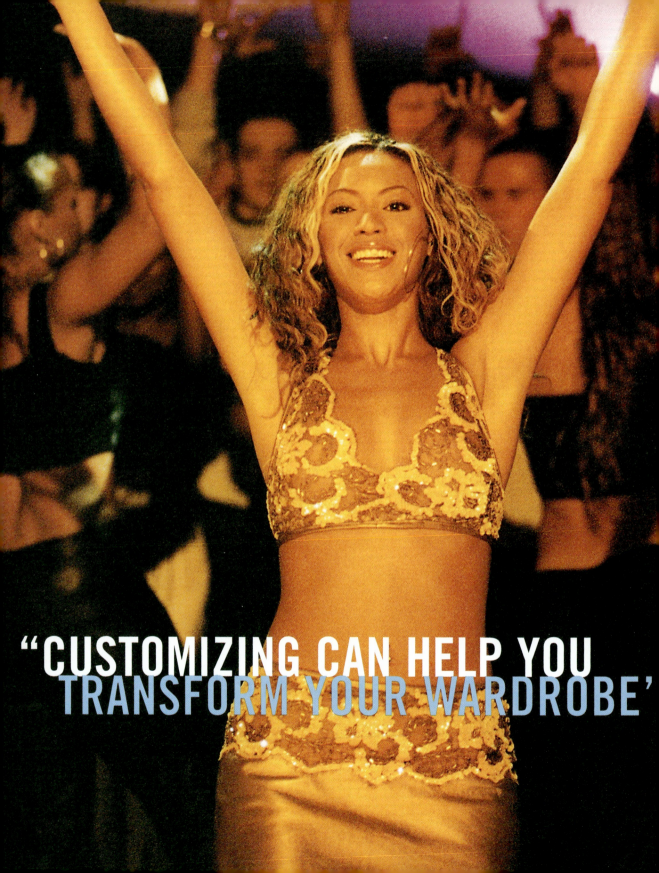

- **Rit dye.** You can use it to dye anything—shoes, pants, underwear, tops. It's available at most drugstores, and it doesn't cost a lot.
- **Spray paint.** We spray-paint jeans and shoes all the time.
- **Scraps of fabric.** I hang on to old scraps of fabric, because I never know when I'll want to use them for customizing. You can slit your jeans on the side and put an insert of fabric on them. That's something easy that anybody can do, and you don't have to buy a big sewing machine to do it.
- **Appliqués.** These are fabrics that come in different images that you apply to jeans, shirts, pillows, or pretty much anything you want. You can make your own by cutting up lace and gluing it on or you can buy them. Appliqués vary in price from less than a dollar to "don't ask." They look really cute on jeans and shirts, which is what I use them on the most. Beyoncé and Solange like adding butterfly appliqués to their jeans.
- **Seam ripper.** A must-have tool for deconstructing clothes. You can buy one at any fabric store.
- **Bleach.** Use bleach to spot your jeans. Or, if you want a more worn-in look, you can use bleach to weaken the denim in spots then poke holes in them using a fork.

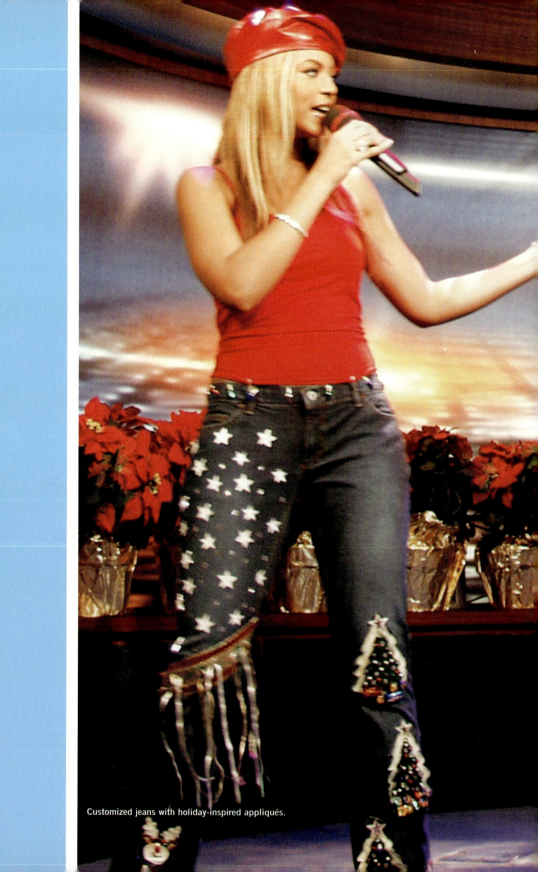

Customized jeans with holiday-inspired appliqués.

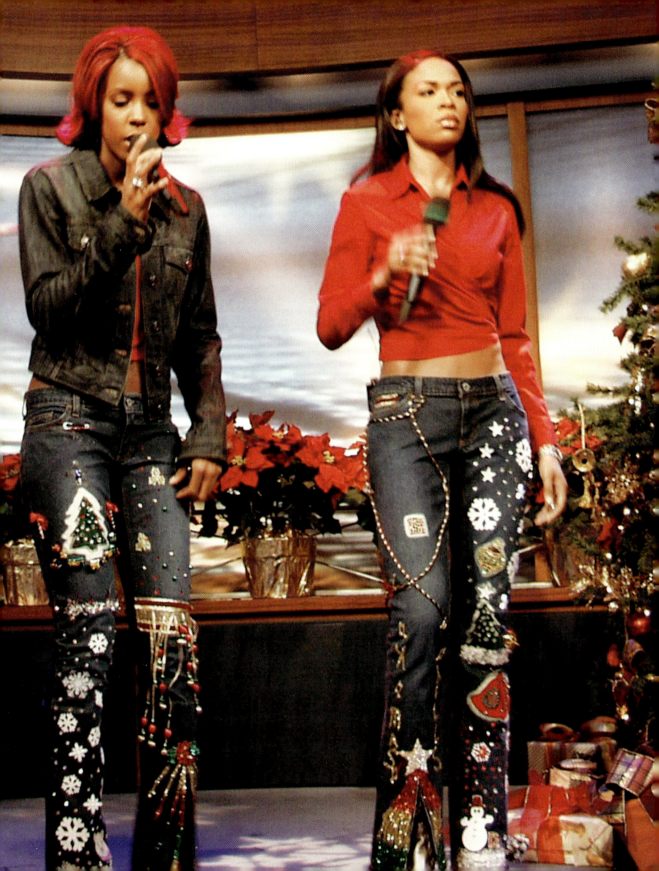

Bootylicious Basics

Follow these fashion tips and everyone will be saying your name.

1. Great-fitting clothes that are in good shape.

Spending the time to find a great, reliable tailor is well worth it for many reasons. If you're not a perfect size "anything," chances are your clothes could use a little cutting and sewing here and there for them to fit your measurements exactly. That's why a good tailor is invaluable. Also, when clothes start to show wear and tear, such as ripped seams or ragged hems, you can call on your tailor to fix them. This way you always look your polished best. If you establish a good relationship with a tailor and let him know that your needs will be ongoing, he'll probably be open to negotiating a price that suits your budget.

2. Work your assets.

Look at yourself and figure out what the best parts of your body are. For Beyoncé, it's her legs. They are long and shapely, so I put her in lots of dresses and skirts to show them off. Kelly has a body that would make you hate her if she wasn't such a great person—she's tall and naturally lean. I think that one of her best assets is her long, regal neck. That's why we've given her a chic short 'do to show it off. I love putting cute necklaces and chokers on her because she carries them off so nicely. Michelle's stomach is her best feature, so I put her in lots of low-slung pants that show off her flat tummy.

3. High heels and thigh-high boots.

No DC outfit would be complete without high-heeled shoes. Thigh-high boots are another classic and important part of their look. When they performed at the 2001 tree-lighting ceremony at Rockefeller Center, Kelly wore a pair of boots that were inspired by the white boots I bought and wore nonstop when I was her age.

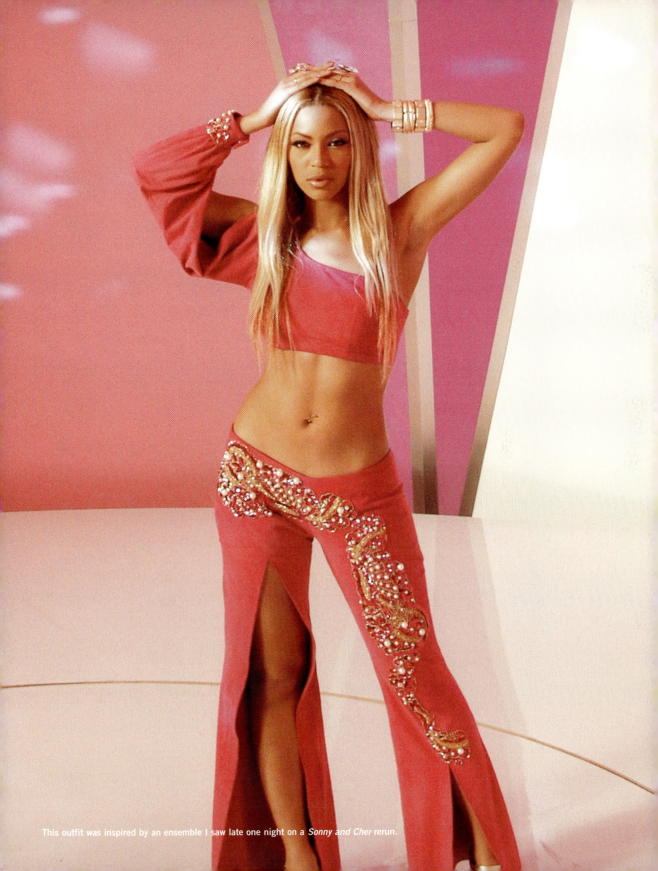

This outfit was inspired by an ensemble I saw late one night on a *Sonny and Cher* rerun.

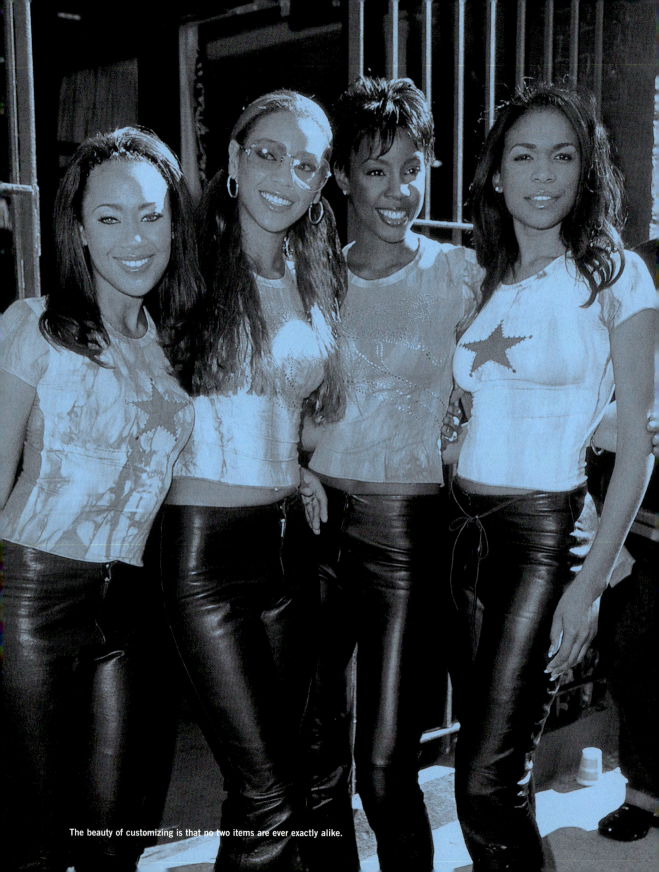
The beauty of customizing is that no two items are ever exactly alike.

4. Bikini top or belly-baring shirt. Every girl needs one in her wardrobe. They look really good with low-slung pants. The trick to wearing little tops is that you need to wear something long on the bottom like a long skirt or hip-hugger pants or else you'll look hootchylicious. Not every girl can wear a bikini top, so the alternative is a belly-baring shirt. If you go the bikini route, just make sure you boobs are not hanging out from under it. Got it?

5. Customized glitter T-shirts. I've always been big on do-it-yourself wardrobes because I love to sew. I realize that not everyone knows how or has the time to sew, but a great way to make your clothing look unique without sewing something from scratch is to get some fabric glue and glitter and start playing. The creative juices will begin flowing in no time.

6. Customized jeans. Jeans are easy to customize by cutting them, deconstructing them, or adding embellishments. Customizing is a great way to "recycle" an old faded pair of jeans that you'd end up tossing. Waste not, want not!

7. Leather pants. A pair of great-fitting, low-slung leather pants are a great addition to any wardrobe. They don't have to be real leather, pleather is fine, and the color is negotiable. Black is the classic color that people buy, but DC has worn pink, red, blue—just about every color under the rainbow. But be sure they fit perfectly. If you're buying ones made of real leather, buy them small, almost too small, because they will stretch.

8. Hats. Beyoncé, Kelly, and Michelle love to wear hats. The pink one that Beyoncé wore in the "Bug A Boo" video became so popular that I saw imitations in many stores all over the world. Michelle likes Kangols, and Kelly likes to wear men's hats.

9. One-shouldered Top. These tops were really big in the eighties and they've come back. I like them because they are sexy and fun. If you've got toned arms, a one-shouldered top is a great way to show them off.

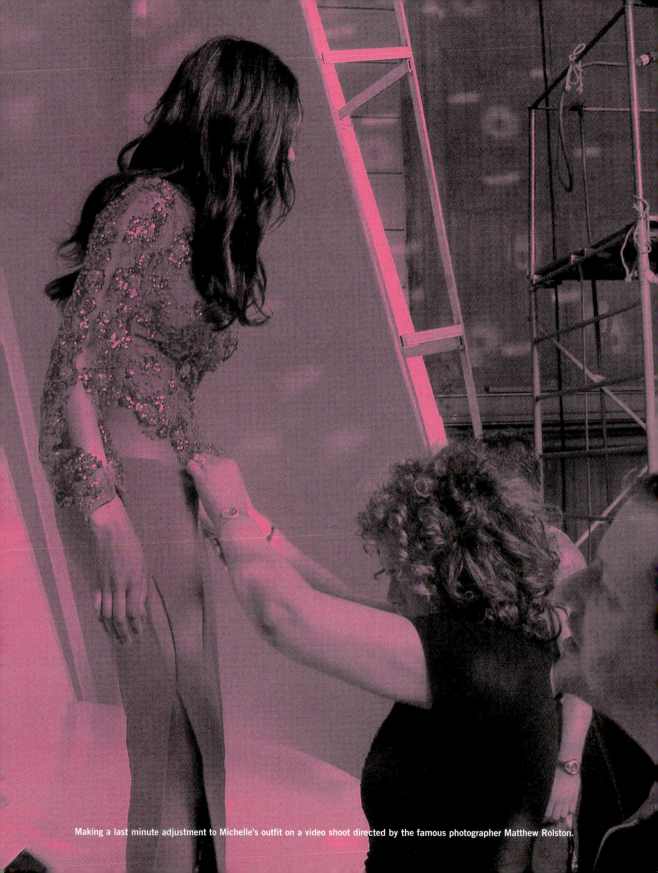

Making a last minute adjustment to Michelle's outfit on a video shoot directed by the famous photographer Matthew Rolston.

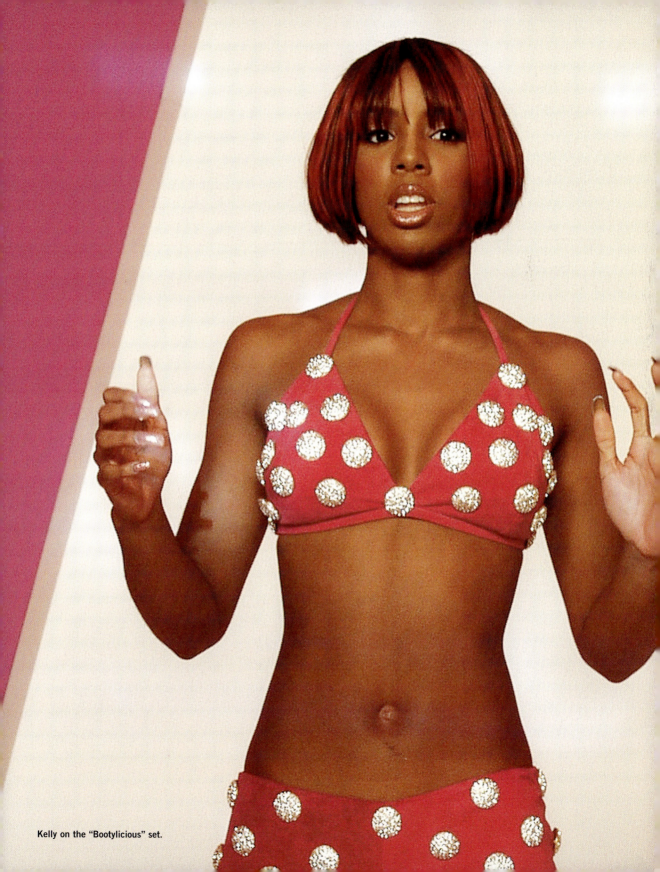
Kelly on the "Bootylicious" set.

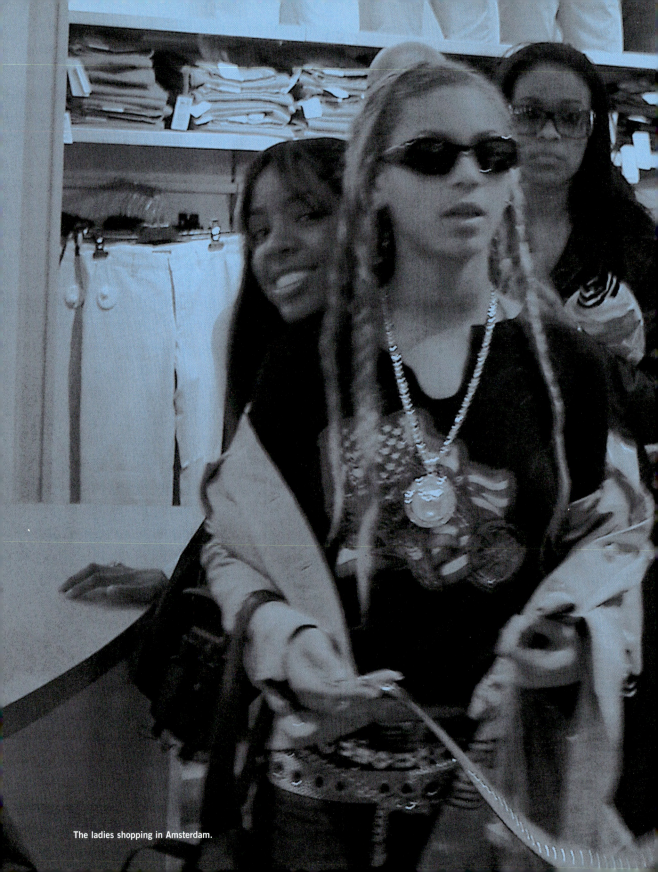
The ladies shopping in Amsterdam.

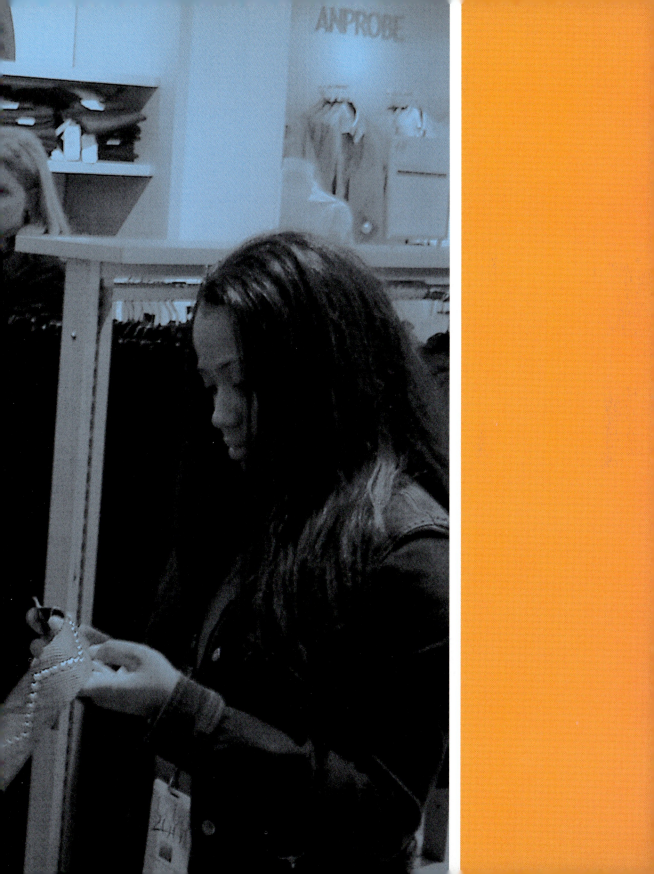

DC FASHION QUIZ

match the girl to her fashion obsession.

1. When she's not performing, she's the classic jeans, blouse, and boots girl.

2. She is obsessed with her shoes matching her bag. Her closet is filled with more than one hundred organized rows of shoes, and right above are rows of corresponding purses that match every pair.

3. Her signature pieces of clothing are the beautiful, tailored designer jackets she loves to splurge on.

4. She is an avid vintage clothes collector.

5. Diamonds aren't her best friend, but they are a close third to her groupmates. She likes to collect small, delicate diamond jewelry like small crosses and bracelets.

6. She likes to wear coats with long tails.

ANSWERS: 1. MICHELLE 2. BEYONCE 3. BEYONCE 4. KELLY 5. KELLY 6. MICHELLE

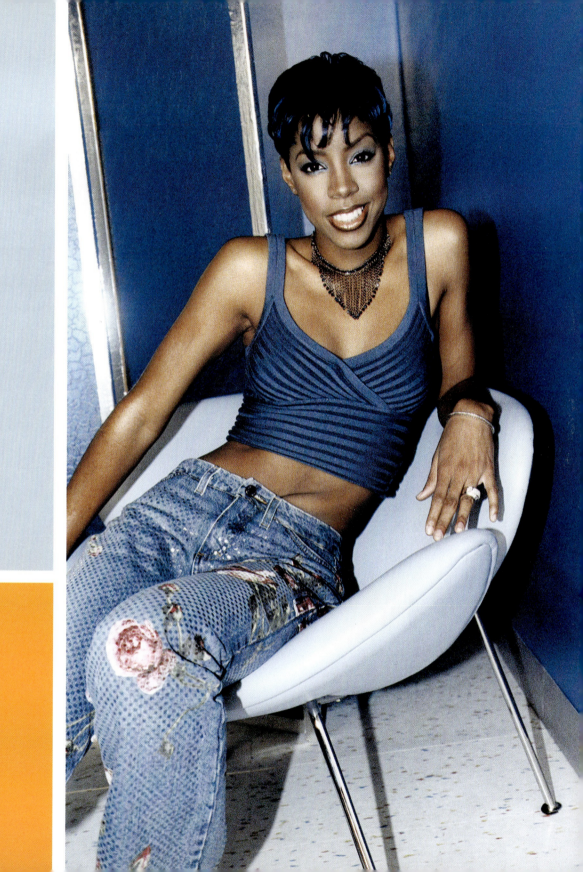

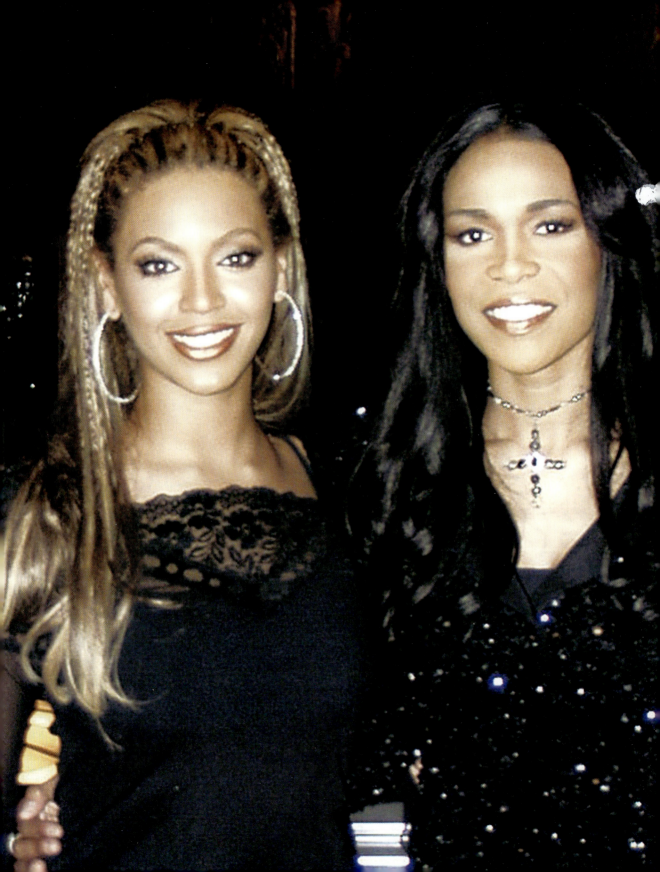

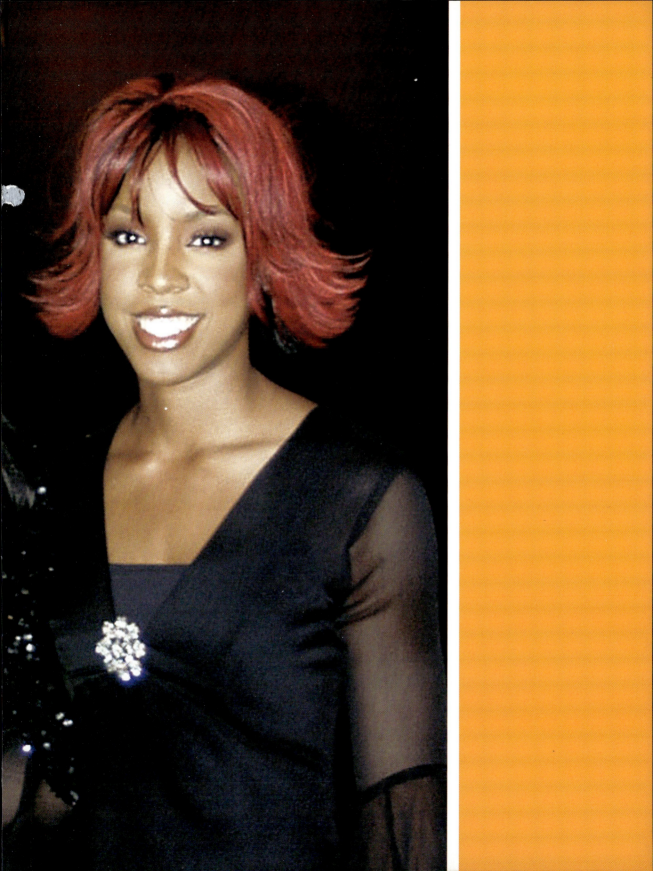

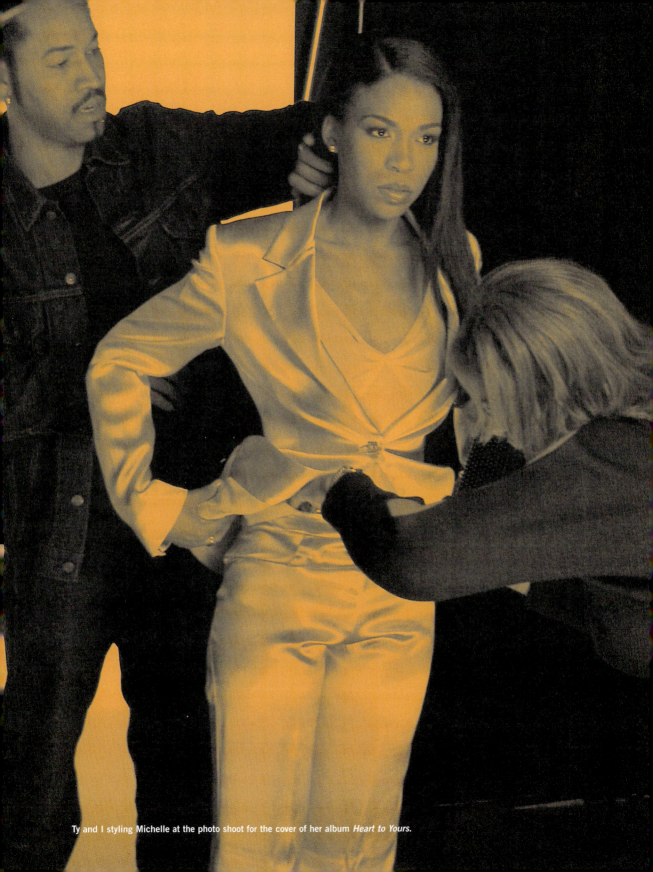

Ty and I styling Michelle at the photo shoot for the cover of her album *Heart to Yours*.

"the girls took their new looks and ran with them"

My salon became the laboratory in which I diva-rized (or, as some people have called it, "Tina-rized") the girls into the ladies they are today—though I can't take all the credit. The girls took their new looks and ran with them—personalizing them in ways I never dreamed. They each have a strong sense of the statement they want to make, and I have a great staff who helps me facilitate it. There were times when we couldn't afford to hire someone to do their hair for an event or photo shoot, so I did their hair in addition to styling them. My assistant, Ty, can also style hair, so between the two of us we've dressed and coiffed all three of them in under three hours! Also, Donna Evans, my top stylist at my salon, helps with styling their hair for video shoots and award shows. She's amazing.

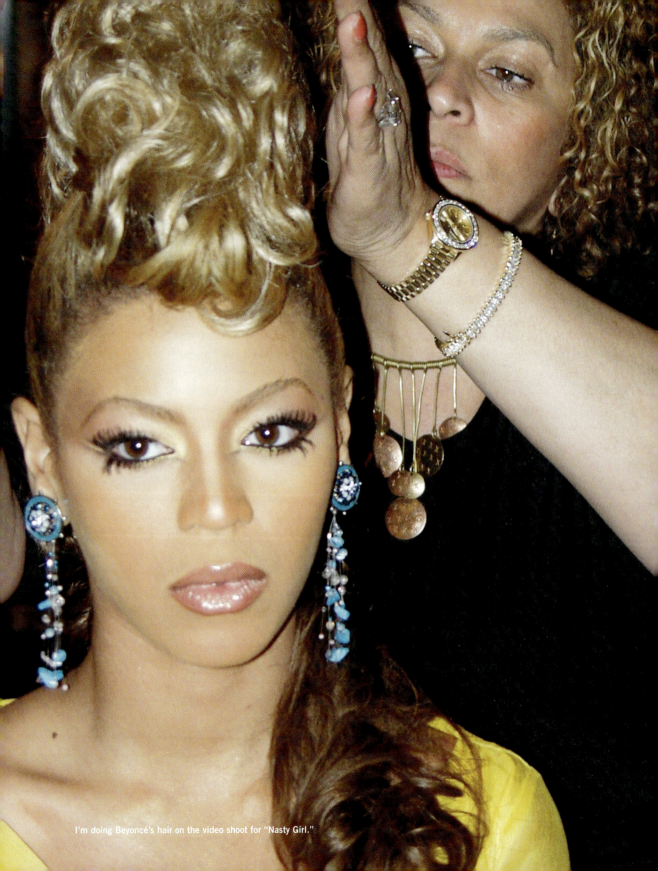

I'm doing Beyoncé's hair on the video shoot for "Nasty Girl."

HAIRSTYLE

Beyoncé grew up running around my hair salon, so she was pretty savvy about the latest beauty trends. She basically came up with all the looks that she's had over the last few years. She's always researching and trying to come up with new techniques for braids and hairstyles, so her hair is constantly changing. She doesn't braid her own hair, but she tells the stylist how she would like it done. People are always asking me about her hair color. For her now famous blond color, we just picked up on her naturally light-brown hair color and started highlighting it more and more using Feria hair dye in Cool Blond.

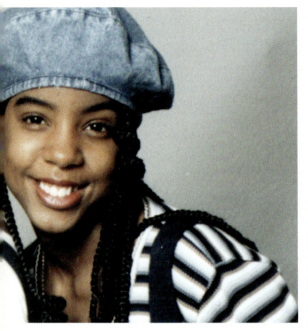

"if you just got a short haircut it would set you apart from every body else"

Kelly's transformation to short hair was striking, because it not only affected the way she looked but her whole attitude changed as well. Her trademark as a little girl was her hair. She was this skinny little wisp of a thing with long braids down her back, and she used to wear corduroys and big shirts all the time. I could tell that lurking behind all her hair was a really pretty face, but I had no idea just how stunning she really was. Beyoncé and I went to work on her around 1996 when Destiny's Child was working on their first album. We told her, "You've got this great face and this cute little figure. If you just got a short haircut it would set you apart from everybody else." It took a lot of courage for Kelly to let me cut her hair because she was only fifteen and didn't know anyone her age who was rockin' a short and sassy 'do. Once she took the plunge and let me cut it, her confidence level rose dramatically.

A few years later she let me talk her into highlighting her hair red. Kelly's fiery red streaks are achieved by highlighting sections of her hair to a light blond, then going over the blond streaks with the color Red Hot by Jazzing. The more times you use the Jazzing, the more vivid the color becomes.

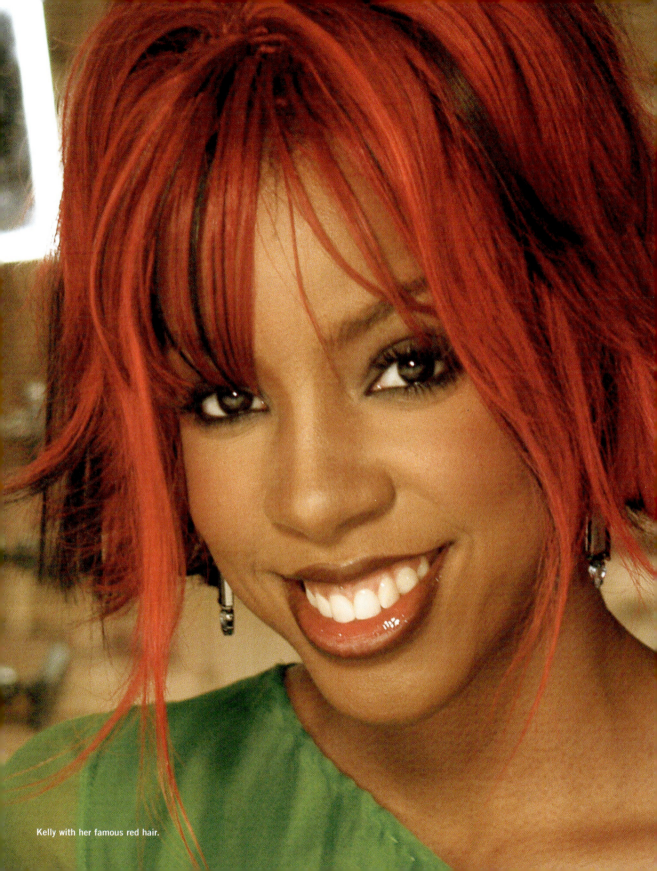

Kelly with her famous red hair.

Michelle's purple hairpieces add a few colorful strands and are a fun and harmless way to experiment with color.

"michelle is a very glamorous woman"

Michelle is a very glamorous woman nowadays, but she'll be the first to tell you that she needed some help in the beginning. She had been a backup singer for the recording artist Monica, and she came to us through a referral from someone who knew we were looking for girls. We asked Michelle to send some pictures of herself, and she emailed a few "glamor shot" pictures that didn't do her any justice. The makeup and hair were wrong, and whoever had done the makeup really overemphasized her eyebrows, which were naturally thick to begin with. Another problem was that she had a mustache. So when we invited her to audition, I first took her to my facialist and had her mustache and eyebrows waxed. At first Michelle joked, "I love my mustache—it's my boyfriend." I said, "Girl, that thing's got to go." After we waxed it, she's never looked back.

Michelle's hair is chemically relaxed. Because that process really dries out the hair, she makes sure she gets a deep conditioning every week. To achieve her hair color, we use Jazzing semipermanent hair color in Eggplant. It's usually applied after the relaxer so it penetrates better. It keeps her hair looking shiny and beautiful.

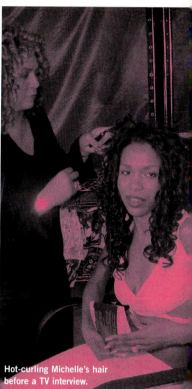

Hot-curling Michelle's hair before a TV interview.

THE STORY OF BEAUTY | 117

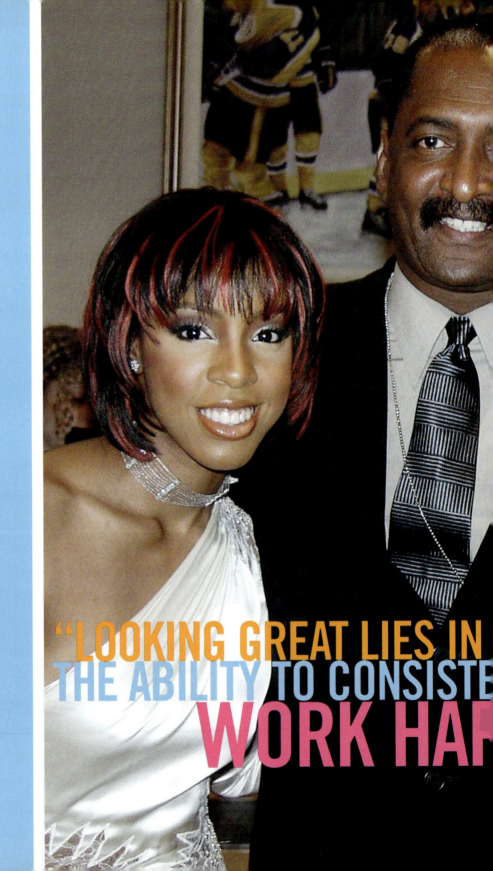

"LOOKING GREAT LIES IN THE ABILITY TO CONSISTE WORK HAR

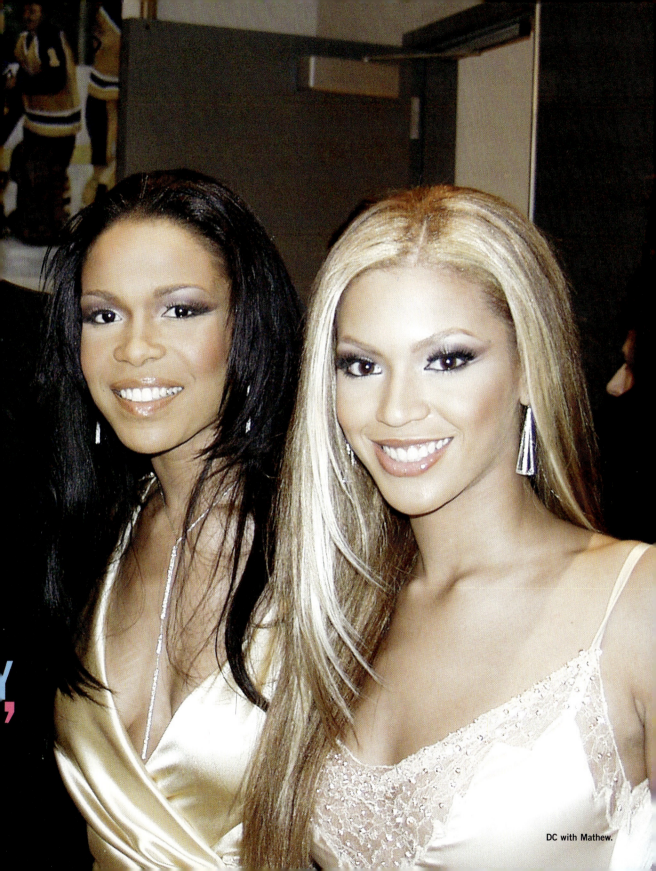

DC with Mathew.

Creating Your Own Bootylicious Hairstyle

If your hair's not right, then you might as well stay home. The secret to having great hair is to take your 'do to whatever extremes you want. Dye it, cut it, crimp it, curl it—just be sure to take care of it. If you dye your hair make sure you condition it properly and keep up with your roots. Every time you blow-dry your hair, use a curling iron, color it, perm it, or relax it, you take some of the protein out. It's important to put that protein back in, so don't try to cut corners with hair care products. If you have to choose between paying extra for a good shampoo or a good deep conditioner, go with the better deep conditioner. Rinsing is one of the most important elements of shiny beautiful hair, so rinse until your hair is squeaky clean.

Hairsprays can wreak havoc on hair. Use products that have very little or no alcohol in them. Don't use aerosol sheen products because they tend to weigh the hair down and contain a lot of alcohol.

Something you should consider incorporating into your hair repertoire is color, and I don't mean just to cover the grays. Use color to make your hair look more alive and in sync with your personality. If you don't want to experiment with permanent color, you can use some of the transparent or semipermanent colors by Cellophane or Jazzing, which give your hair a glow of color and wash out in a few shampoos. (A word of warning: If you have light hair and go too much darker than your natural hair color, it won't completely wash out.) Highlights are another great way to color your hair without too much damage.

Poorly maintained hair is never hot. A good haircut is essential. Be sure to get it trimmed every six weeks, and you shouldn't go to just anybody or look in the Yellow Pages. Do your homework. Don't be afraid to stop anyone you see with a great haircut and ask her where she got it done and which stylist did it. That last bit is important—it's not the salon that makes a haircut, it's the stylist. Not every stylist at a salon has equal ability. Even if you have to save money for your hair service, it's well worth the wait. After all, if your hair looks healthy and sharp, you can throw on a pair of jeans and still look fabulous.

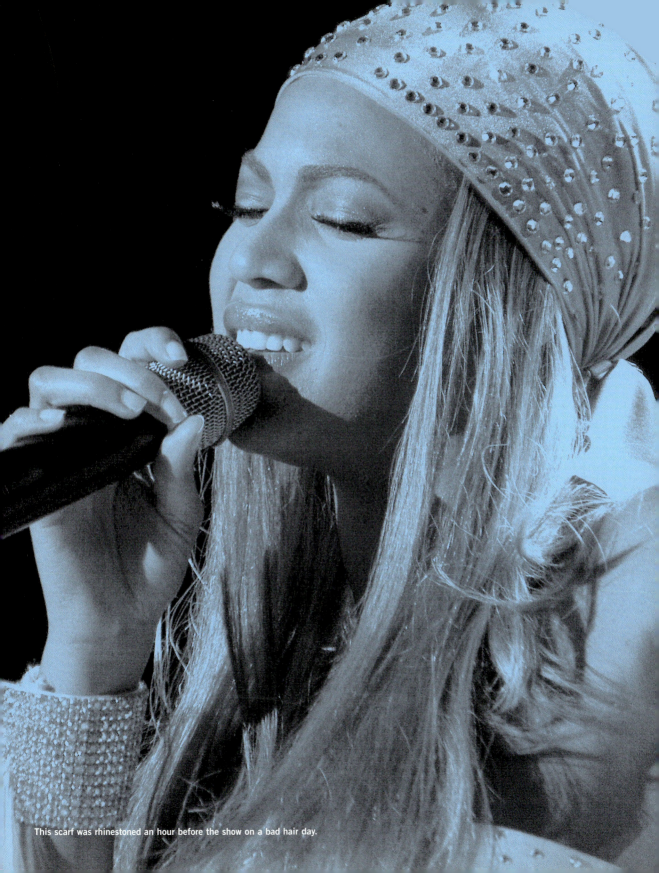

This scarf was rhinestoned an hour before the show on a bad hair day.

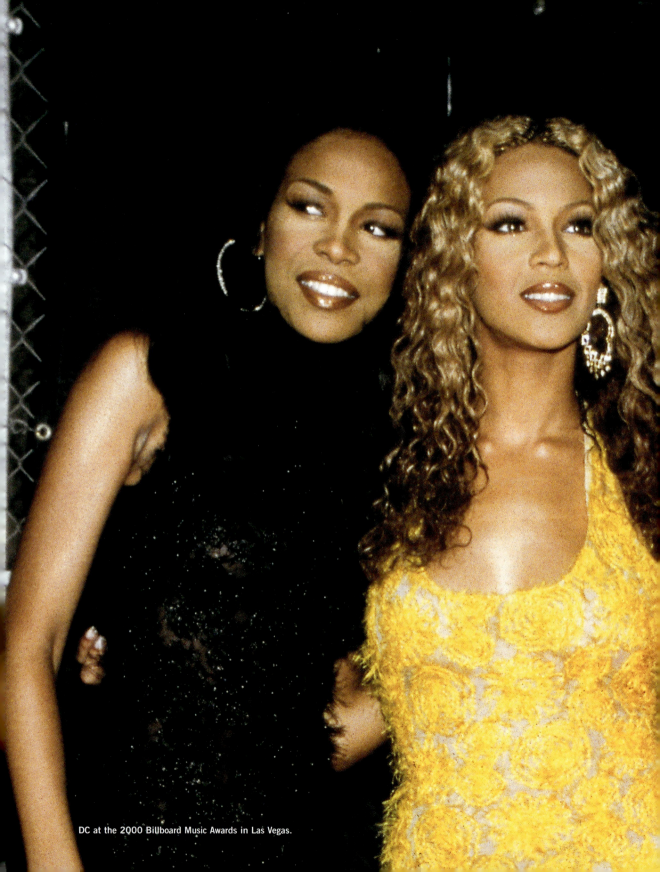

DC at the 2000 Billboard Music Awards in Las Vegas.

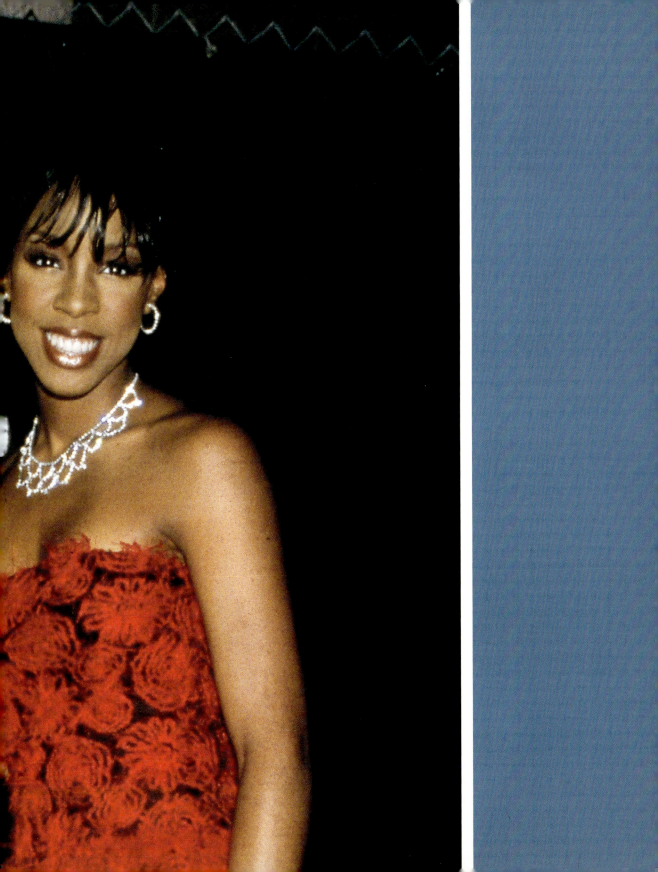

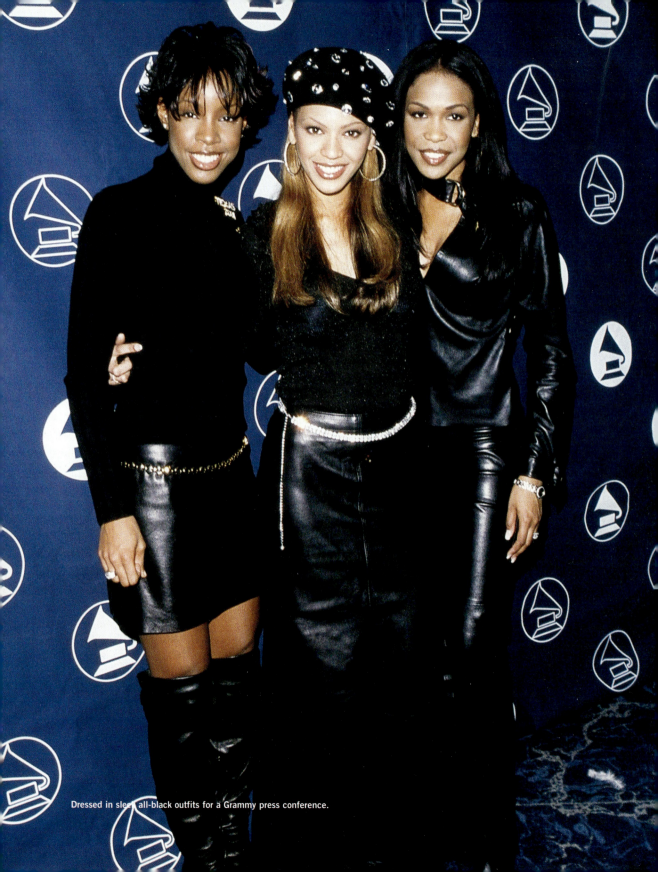

Dressed in sleek all-black outfits for a Grammy press conference.

GIVING GOOD FACE

LIKE MOST PEOPLE, WHEN BEYONCÉ, KELLY, OR MICHELLE FEEL BAD ON THE INSIDE, IT AFFECTS THEIR OUTER BEAUTY AS WELL. THEY ALL HANDLE STRESS AND DISAPPOINTMENT DIFFERENTLY, BUT THE OUTCOME ON THEIR LOOKS IS THE SAME ACROSS THE BOARD. THAT'S WHEN THEIR SKIN DOESN'T GLOW, THEIR HAIR DOESN'T SHINE, AND THEIR THOUSAND-WATT SMILES NEED NEW LIGHTBULBS. ONE COMMON MISCONCEPTION PEOPLE HAVE ABOUT CELEBRITIES IS THAT THEY AREN'T "REAL" PEOPLE. THE FACT IS, ALL THE GIRLS IN DC ARE VERY REAL YOUNG WOMEN—THEY JUST HAPPEN TO BE LIVING IN EXTRAORDINARY CIRCUMSTANCES. JUST LIKE EVERYONE ELSE, THEY SUFFER HEARTBREAK, BOUTS OF DEPRESSION, AND LOW SELF-ESTEEM. ABOVE ANYTHING ELSE THEY ARE GIRLS WHO ARE FIGURING THINGS OUT AS THEY GO, JUST LIKE THE REST OF US.

I've always believed that the formula for happiness, success, and looking great lies in the ability to consistently work hard, be disciplined, and shut out negativity. It's common sense, and nothing new to many successful people. Because of Mathew's background in sales, these are values he's learned over the years, and we reinforce them in the girls. My husband and I have come under fire because we encourage these values. The "haters" have said many hurtful and unprintable things about the whole Destiny's Child family. Some have been quick to dismiss the ladies' talent as singers by saying, "Well, they're pretty girls who got lucky." Sure, they are pretty, but so are lots of girls. The things that set Destiny's Child apart are their talent and their unshakable confidence. Through hard work and shutting out negativity we have all been able to overcome the hardships we've faced. When you feel good and are doing something with your life that is rewarding to your mind, body, and soul, it's not that hard to look beautiful.

Success, No Stress, and Lots of Happiness

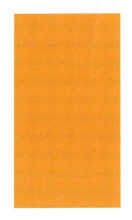

We've all had bad days. When the band was under stress and had uncertainties in the group, Beyoncé had major acne. She was given medicine, pills, injections by her dermatologist, and nothing worked. She was distraught over what was happening with the group and her skin problems made her feel worse. When your face is a mess it affects everything you do. Your self-esteem is low, so it affects your body language, which affects how people view you, which indirectly affects how you're treated. The ladies get photographed so often and so much of their career is tied into image that there is pressure to keep their faces looking clear. That leads to more stress, which leads to more pimples. When Beyoncé's face broke out, it made her depression over the problems in the group even worse. On top of it, there was a very real possibility that the group wouldn't be able to go on with only her and Kelly left. When she finally got tired of feeling so bad, she was inspired to pick up her journals and start writing to clear her mind. She started praying for guidance. Once she allowed herself to be guided by her faith, she felt the anxiety lift and her face began to clear up. The key to beauty is inner peace, and inner peace is found by keeping your mind free of worry. We all know this can be hard, but we need to try.

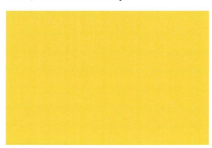

Beyoncé resting on the set of "Emotions." Remember that drinking lots of water is the key to looking bootylicious.

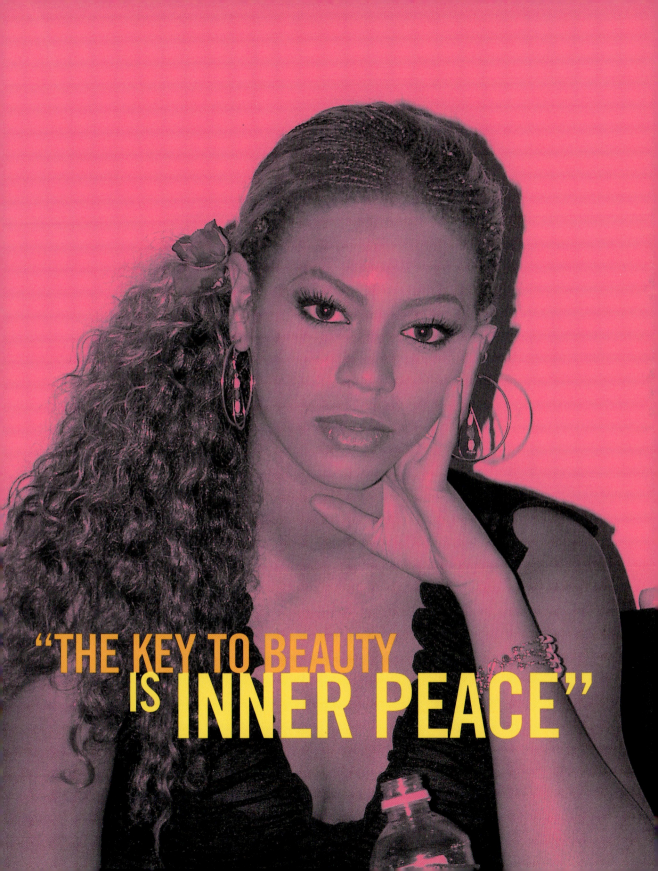

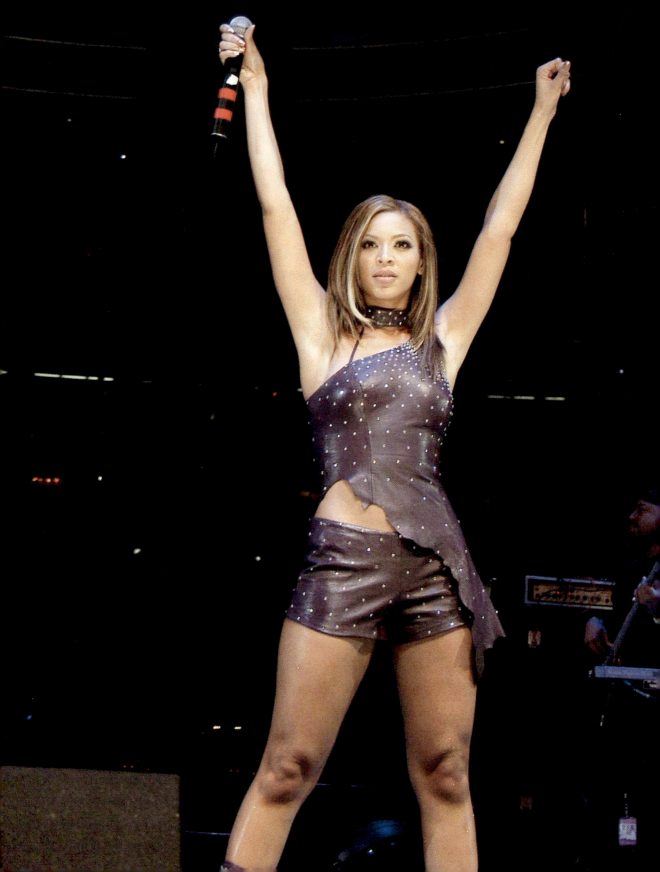

THE DOS AND DON'TS OF KEEPING A SURVIVOR'S FRAME OF MIND:

1. **Do stand up straight.** Standing tall generates optimism.

2. **Don't get involved in "pity parties."** Don't get caught up with people who complain about everything and constantly see things in a negative light. These people will only bring you down.

3. **Do grow up and face the facts.** It's called maturity and being a woman. Certain things just aren't meant to happen. You aren't going to have that same figure you had at sixteen ever again. You may not end up with that great guy you went out with last week who hasn't called since.

4. **Don't let a boyfriend make you feel bad about your body.** If he loves your body the way it is, then he's a keeper. If he lowers your self-esteem by not accepting your body, then you need to dismiss him and find someone who loves you just the way you are.

5. **Do exercise for health purposes and don't obsess about monitoring every pound and inch.** Part of being bootylicious is loving your body no matter what kind of shape you have. Accentuate the positives, take care of your health, and don't fret over not being a size 6. It ain't no thing—really, it's not.

6. **When setbacks occur, give yourself time to grieve.** As Aaliyah sang, "Dust yourself off and try again."

7. **Don't buy clothes that cause you drama.** This means don't buy a pair of pants that you can't wear until you "lose a few pounds," or skirts so short you can't sit down, or clothes that are so sheer and tight you feel self-conscious and physically stifled.

8. **Do your own thing.** Everyone is given different gifts, so don't focus on someone else's. Find your natural talents and use them well. People will notice and you'll be happier.

9. **Do love yourself.** It's a fact of life that there are going to be people who make you feel bad about yourself or don't like you—the "haters." They try to take the wind out of your sails when something good happens to you. If you love yourself then the "haters" won't matter, because you realize that their "stank" attitude is their problem, not yours. There is a song that Solange wrote called "This Song's For You." She wrote it after someone told her she wasn't going to do well because she was Beyoncé's little sister. The lyrics contain her own personal mantra that she uses to pump herself up. It goes, "Say to yourself, I rock. I'm hot. I'm not gonna stop. Now go." The great thing about affirmations is that you can repeat them to yourself whenever you're feeling blue. They can really work to lift you out of a funky mood.

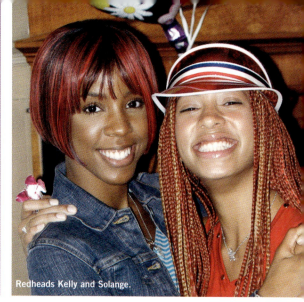
Redheads Kelly and Solange.

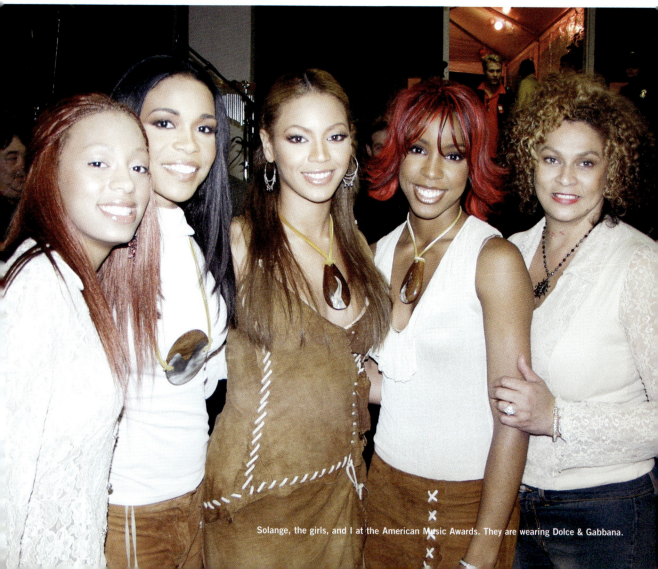
Solange, the girls, and I at the American Music Awards. They are wearing Dolce & Gabbana.

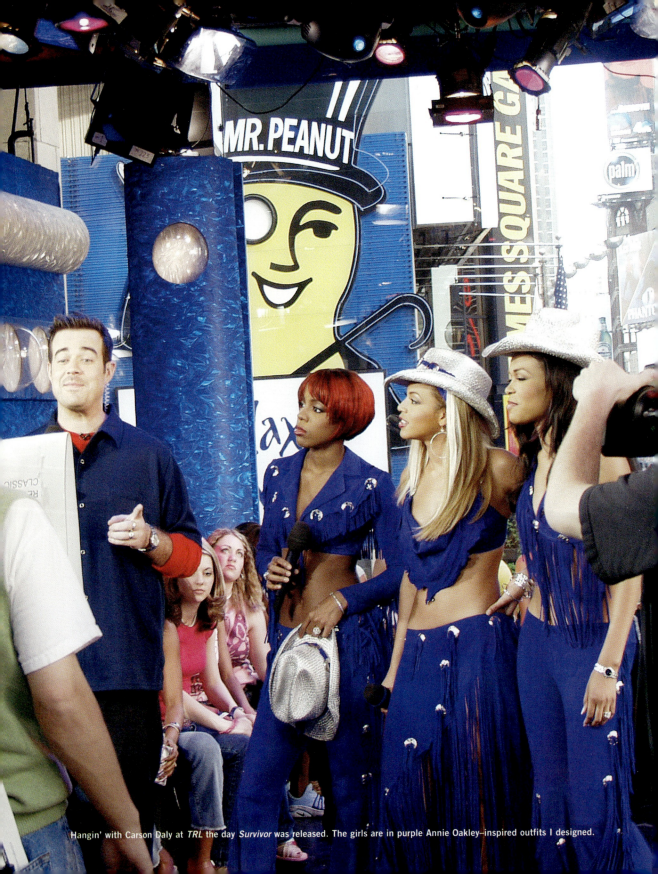

Hangin' with Carson Daly at *TRL* the day *Survivor* was released. The girls are in purple Annie Oakley–inspired outfits I designed.

SHOW TIME

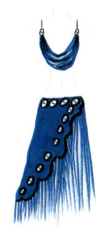

THE TIME EQUATION FOR DC'S HAIR AND MAKEUP BEFORE A SHOW OR TV APPEARANCE IS USUALLY ONE HOUR PER GIRL. ONLY UNDER THE BEST OF CIRCUMSTANCES DO WE USUALLY GET THIS LONG TO GET THE GIRLS READY. THAT'S WHY IT'S A GOOD THING THAT I'VE HAD SO MANY DIFFERENT CAREERS. I'VE OWNED A BEAUTY SALON IN HOUSTON FOR TWELVE YEARS, PUBLISHED THE HAIR MAGAZINE *SALON INTERNATIONAL*, AND WAS A MAKEUP REP FOR SHISEIDO AND A BEAUTICIAN FOR YEARS. SO I OFTEN DO THE GIRLS' HAIR IN ADDITION TO THEIR WARDROBE, WHICH SAVES US TIME.

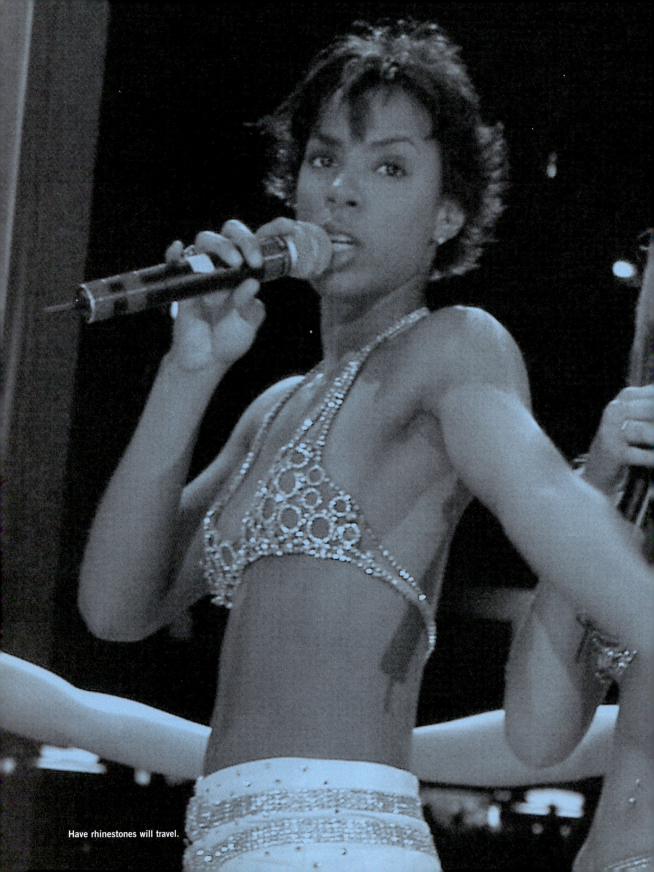

Have rhinestones will travel.

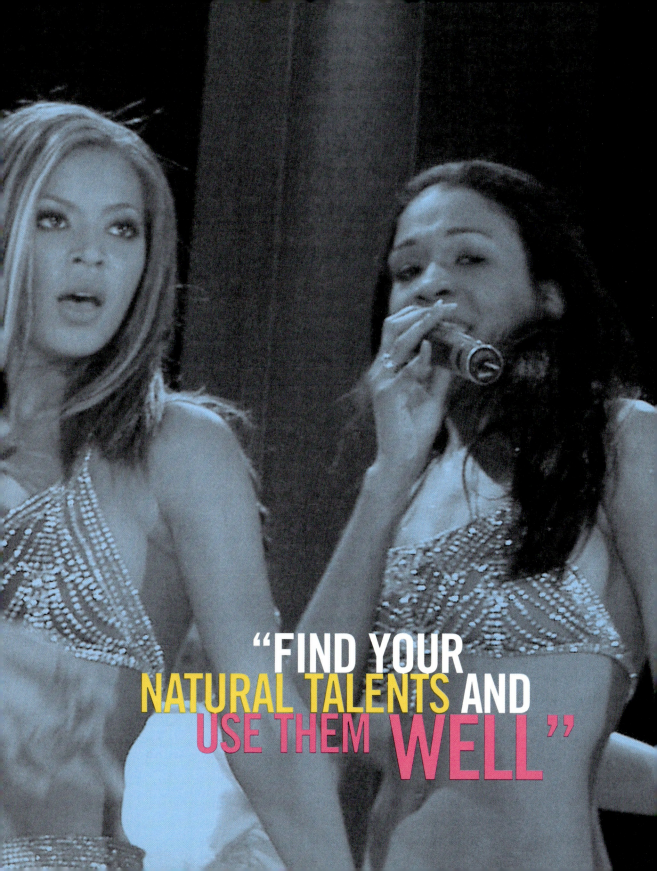

Unveiling their Hasbro dolls. I designed the outfits the dolls are wearing.

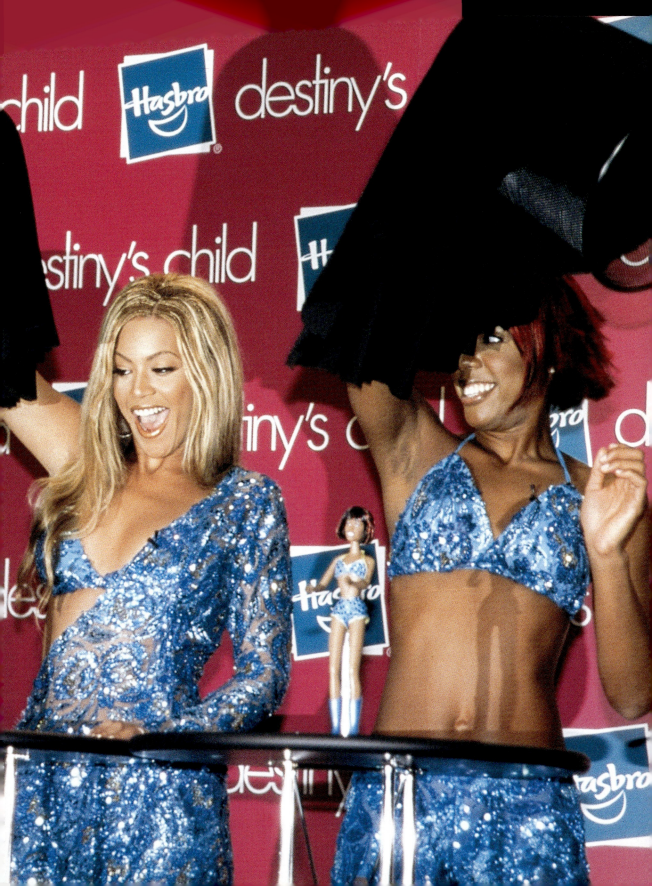

"makeup artists know exactly how to make the girls' faces look bootylicious"

With the schedule that DC keeps, we are truly blessed to have two makeup artists who consistently work with us and know exactly how to make the girls' faces look bootylicious, regardless of how little sleep they've had or whether one of their faces has broken out. Reggie Wells is a wonderful makeup artist and has done makeup for all the great divas, from Aretha Franklin to Whitney Houston to supermodel Iman, as well as the flawless Diahann Carroll. He was Oprah Winfrey's makeup artist for a long time and still does her makeup for her magazine covers. It's an honor to have him as the girls' makeup artist. Billy B. worked with DC for two and a half years and still does when his schedule permits. He is in demand doing the makeup for beautiful young artists such as Mary J. Blige, Missy Elliott, and Pink. Both Reggie and Billy have become like family, and we cherish our time with them. They know the girls' makeup preferences and know how to apply their makeup in a way that will last through lights, sweating, and quick costume changes.

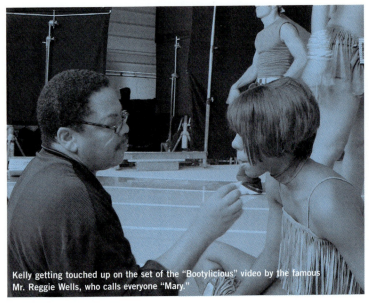

Kelly getting touched up on the set of the "Bootylicious" video by the famous Mr. Reggie Wells, who calls everyone "Mary."

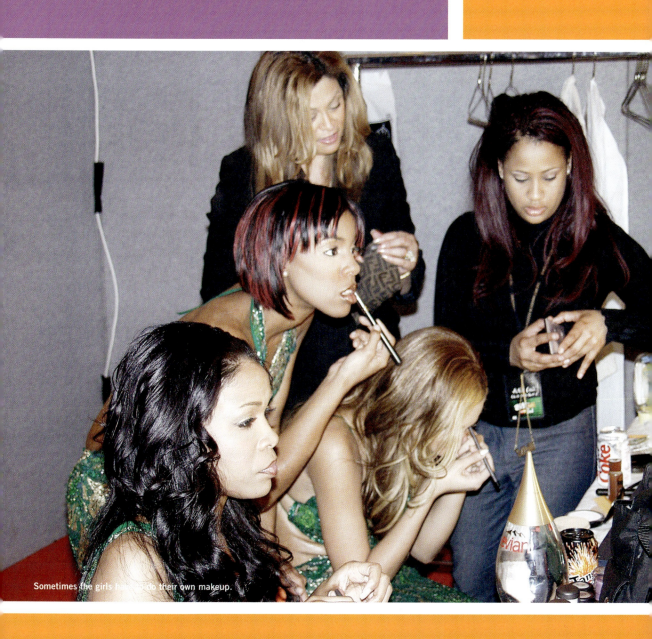

Sometimes the girls have to do their own makeup.

Beyoncé likes a fresh-looking sheen on her skin and really hates wearing heavy foundation, so Reggie loves to dramatize her eyes. He strokes light brown shadow along the whole upper lid and a darker shade in the crease and the lower lash line. He also bleached her eyebrows to match her blond hair. Billy B. loves to add a hint of gold or bronze to her face to make it really glow and play up her natural skin tone.

Kelly loves lip gloss so Reggie and Billy B. always know to have a tube handy for her. She also likes wild colors, so Reggie uses high-watt colors like electric blue on her eyes. She's the rocker chick of the bunch, so for a glam-rock look he'll use red cream eye shadow to match her red hair color.

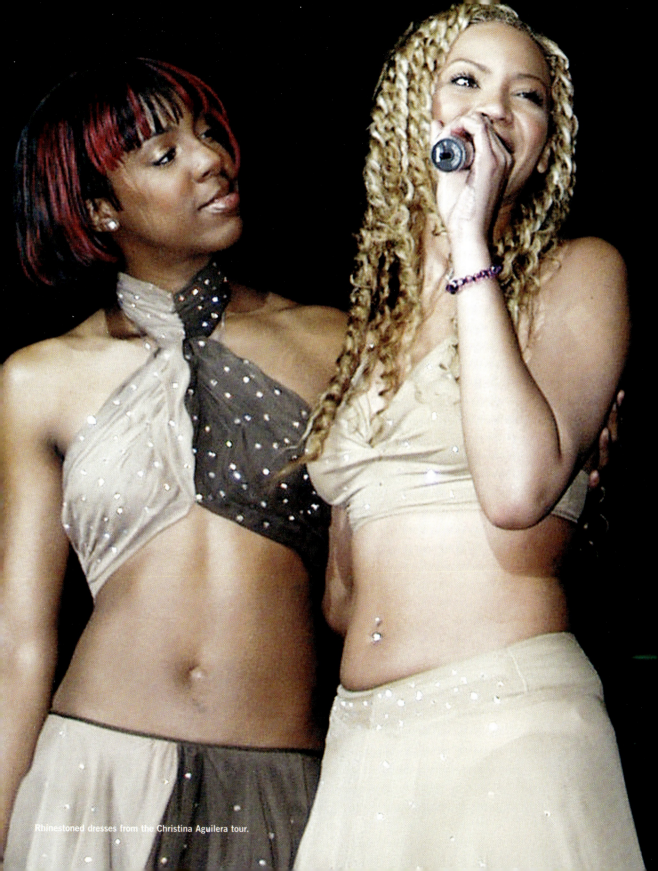

Rhinestoned dresses from the Christina Aguilera tour.

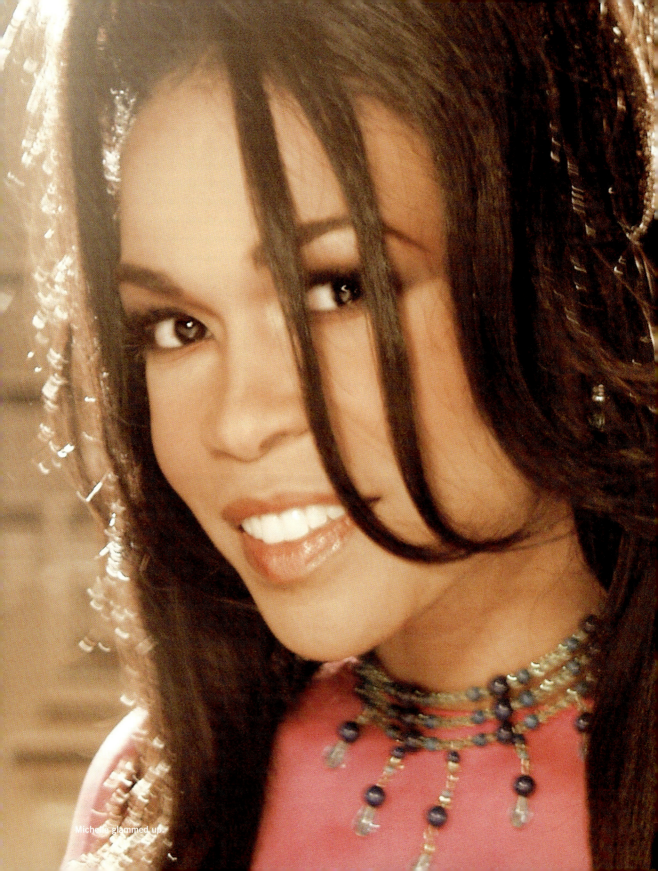
Michelle glammed up.

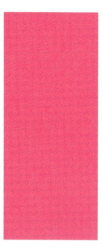

Michelle is the experimental one in the group when it comes to makeup. She has great features, but she has to be careful not to wear too much eye makeup because her eyes are small. A lot of makeup tends to close up small eyes. That's why Reggie steers clear of dark eye colors for her. He sticks to subtle eye shadows like pastels and earth tones, which he extends all the way out to her temples.

Makeup artists are an integral part of an entertainer's life, and it's important to get the best. However, there are things nonentertainers can do to look like superstars. First, start by going to an upscale department store or M·A·C makeup counter. Find a salesperson who is wearing great natural-looking makeup and ask her to do a makeover on you. If you love your new look, buy the basics in the colors she used on you. The basics include foundation, concealer, blush, and powder. These are the important items you shouldn't skimp on. You also should invest in good makeup brushes. It's okay to go the inexpensive route on eye shadow, mascara, eyeliner, and lipstick. They can be bought at the drugstore and work just as well as their expensive counterparts.

BEAUTY IS OUR BAG!

WE TRAVEL ALL OVER THE WORLD AND THERE ARE CERTAIN PRODUCTS THAT THE LADIES NEVER LEAVE HOUSTON WITHOUT. M·A·C LIPGLASS IS KELLY'S HANDS-DOWN PERSONAL FAVORITE. SHE CAN'T GET ENOUGH OF THE STUFF. SHE'S ALWAYS ASKING, "WHERE'S MY GLASS?" AS SHE ZOOMS BY THE MAKEUP CHAIR ON HER WAY TO THE STAGE. FALSE EYELASHES ARE A MUST, AND MICHELLE ESPECIALLY LOVES TO EXPERIMENT WITH THEM. SHE TRIES ALL DIFFERENT STYLES AND COLORS. ANY DRUGSTORE VERSION WILL DO, JUST PRACTICE PUTTING THEM ON SO YOU AREN'T WALKING AROUND LOOKING CRAZY WITH YOUR FALSE LASHES HANGING CROOKED. THAT'S NOT CUTE. EYE CREAM IS ESSENTIAL. MY DAUGHTER SOLANGE IS ONLY SIXTEEN AND SHE ALWAYS DABS EYE CREAM ON BEFORE BED. SHE'S SO HOOKED ON IT THAT SHE'S GOTTEN THE OTHER GIRLS TO USE IT, BUT THEY AREN'T ALWAYS AS DISCIPLINED AS SHE IS. BEYONCÉ, WHO WE ALL GET ON FOR NOT ALWAYS TAKING HER MAKEUP OFF BEFORE BED, SAYS, "I THINK IT'S TOO LATE FOR US TO START USING EYE CREAM. WE SHOULD HAVE BEEN ON EYE CREAM AT TWELVE." TO WHICH I SAY, "YES, BUT IT'S NEVER TOO LATE TO START A GOOD HABIT." ONE THING THAT EVERY WOMAN IN THE FAMILY WEARS IS L'ORÉAL VOLUMINOUS MASCARA. TWO COATS WILL HAVE YOU LOOKING BRIGHT-EYED AND BUSHY-TAILED EVEN IF YOU'RE ONLY OPERATING ON THREE HOURS OF SLEEP.

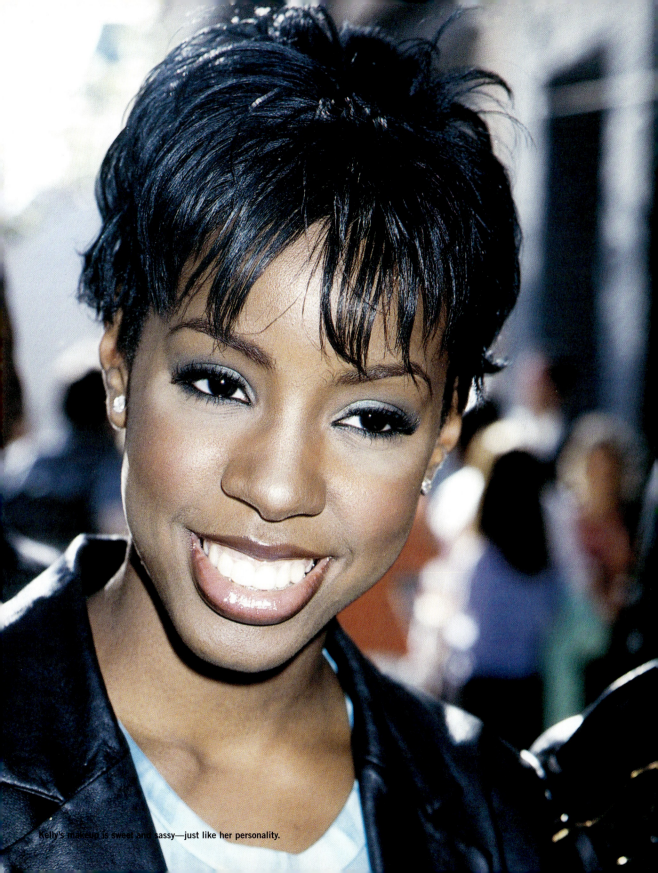
Kelly's makeup is sweet and sassy—just like her personality.

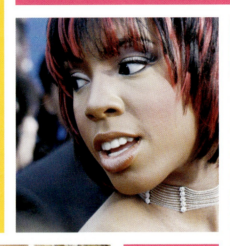
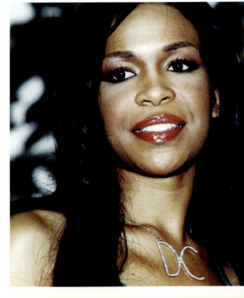
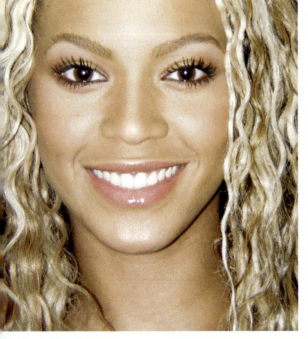

DOIN' LASHES DC STYLE

PUTTING ON FALSE LASHES CAN BE TRICKY THE FIRST TIME, BUT WITH A LITTLE PRACTICE YOU'LL BE ABLE TO PUT THEM ON WITH NO PROBLEM. HERE'S A QUICK TUTORIAL.

1. Put your eye shadow and eyeliner on, and put mascara on your own lashes.

2. Peel the lash strip gently away from the platform and hold it against your own lash. It should start about a quarter-inch from the inside corner of your eye and end with your natural lash line.

3. The trick to false lashes is the fit. If the lash strip is too long, use scissors to cut off the extra length at the outer edge.

4. Hold the strip by one end and run a thin one line of the lash adhesive along the base of the lashes. (A good tool to spread the glue is the round end of a bobby pin.)

5. Hold the lash strip by both ends and flex it back and forth, forming the shape of a horseshoe.

6. Look down into a mirror on your bathroom counter or dressing table and place the lash as close as possible to your lash roots.

7. Press the ends into place with the rounded end of a bobby pin—but not the pin that has the glue on it.

8. Let the glue dry and carefully apply mascara as needed to comb and blend your natural lashes with the false ones.

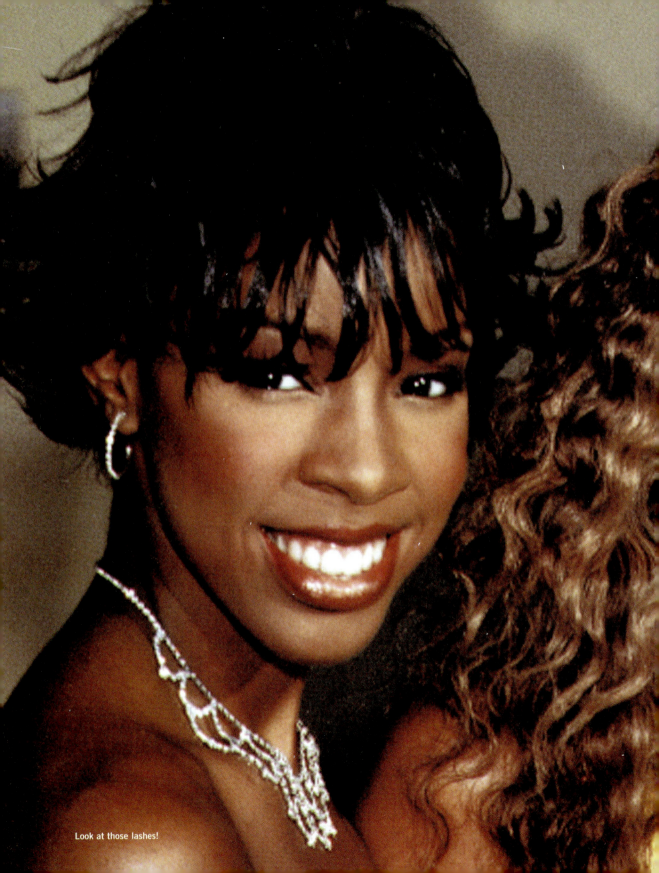

Look at those lashes!

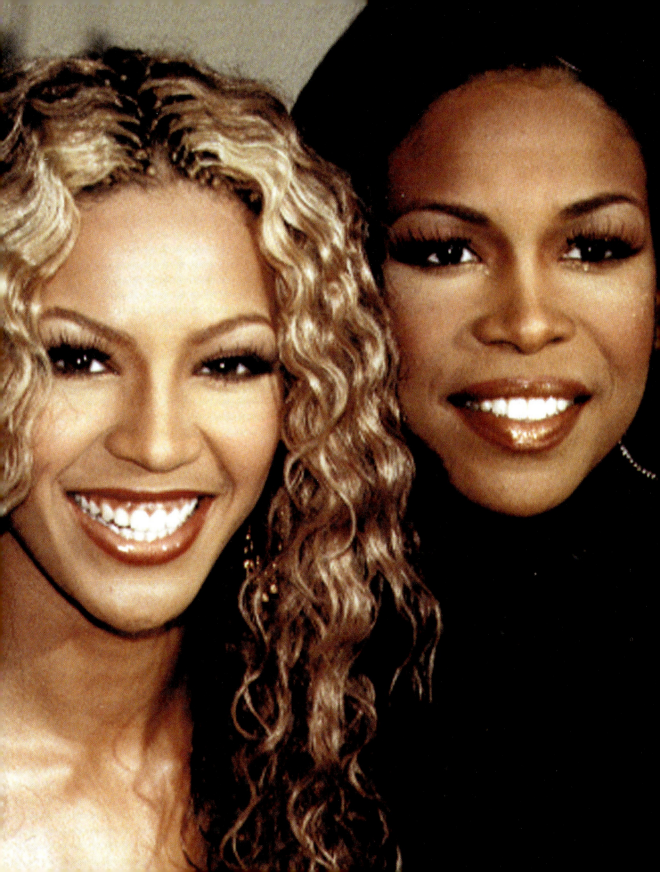

DC Maintenance Routine

A lot of showbiz beauty is all about smoke and mirrors, so it's unfair for people to compare themselves to the stars they see on TV. I know it seems like a lot of celebrity women are born with almost unreal beauty, but what showbiz people almost never tell you is that it usually takes a village to make stars look as glamorous as they do. Since most people don't have a team of experts to put their face on them, here are a few pointers the DC girls use. You can incorporate these into your beauty routine to cultivate a superstar look of your own.

Arch those eyebrows. You'll be surprised what a dramatic difference something so simple can make. This is something you shouldn't try to attempt yourself the first time. Get a professional to do it initially and then, if you think you're handy with tweezers, just maintain the shape by picking strays as they grow back.

Eliminate facial hair. If Michelle can do it, so can you. It's quick and relatively painless. There are do-it-yourself home waxing kits that can be purchased for a song at the drugstore. Or you can opt to have a professional do it. If it's just a mustache or eyebrows, it shouldn't cost more than $5 to $10 dollars each depending on how chi-chi the salon is. If you are waxing more, it can get pricey. Tell the facialist ahead of time what you need waxed, and she may give you a cheaper rate than getting everything waxed separately.

Wear lots of color on your face. Don't fall into the trap of wearing the same black eyeliner and neutral lip color every day. Jazz it up! Experiment with wearing different and interesting colors on your face that you might not normally wear. Warning! If you get jiggy with the eye makeup then ease up and go neutral on the lip color and vice versa. Too much drama on eyes *and* lips takes your look straight to Hootchyville. Don't go there!

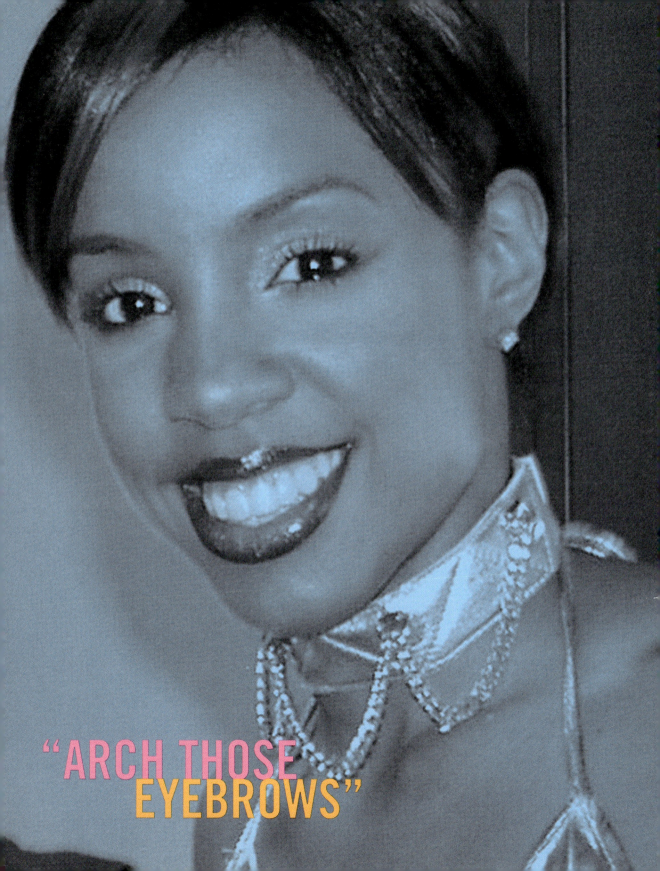

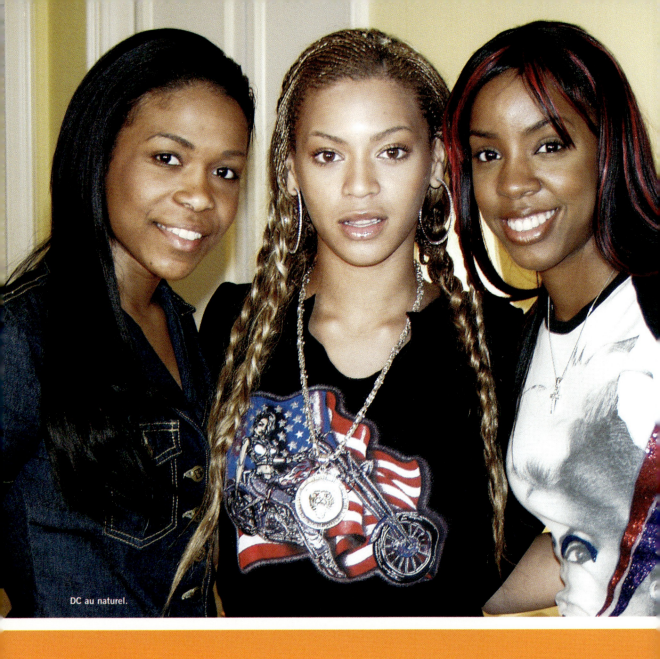

DC au naturel.

DC'S BEDTIME BEAUTY RITUALS

GREAT MAKEUP CAN ONLY DO SO MUCH. NOTHING CAN WORK MIRACLES, SO IT'S IMPORTANT TO TAKE CARE OF YOUR SKIN. WHERE THE MAKEUP ENDS, GOOD HABITS BEGIN.

1. ***Take your makeup off.*** Beyoncé sometimes slacks in this department, but Kelly and Michelle are very disciplined about taking their makeup off before bed. Do it. It's important.

2. ***Pray or meditate.*** When you're stressed, it affects your looks, your attitude, and the way you treat yourself and others. So if you have a lot on your mind, praying, meditating, or both can help you deal with all the things troubling you so you don't have to be weighed down by them anymore. If you're not stressed, use prayer or meditation to count your blessings.

3. ***Wear a silk scarf to protect your hair.*** Yes, the scarf should be silk. This is great for keeping your 'do in check while you're asleep. The other benefit is that your pillowcase won't rub all the natural oils out of your hair while you sleep, which is especially helpful if you have dry hair to begin with, which all the DC girls have because of heat elements and hot lights.

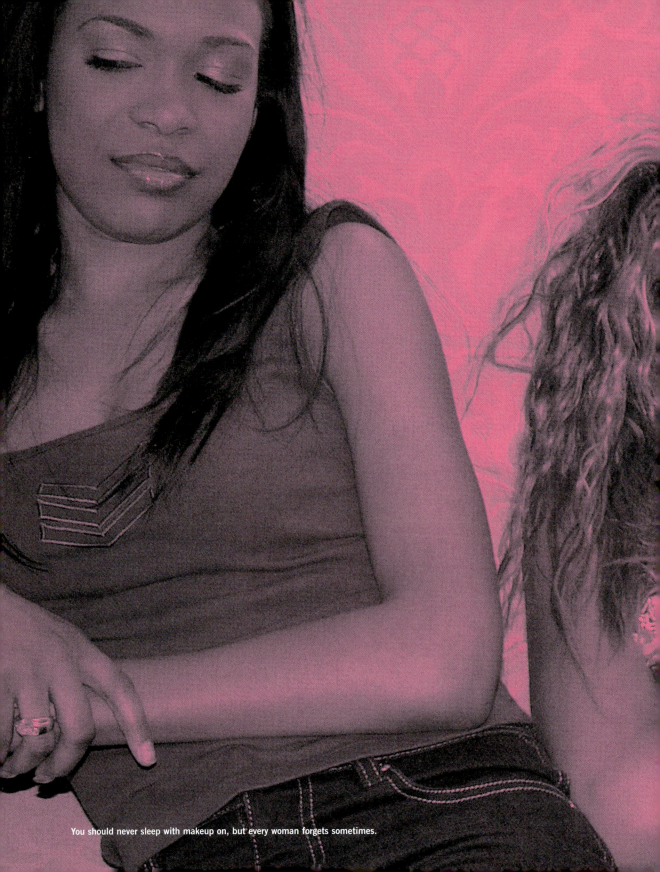

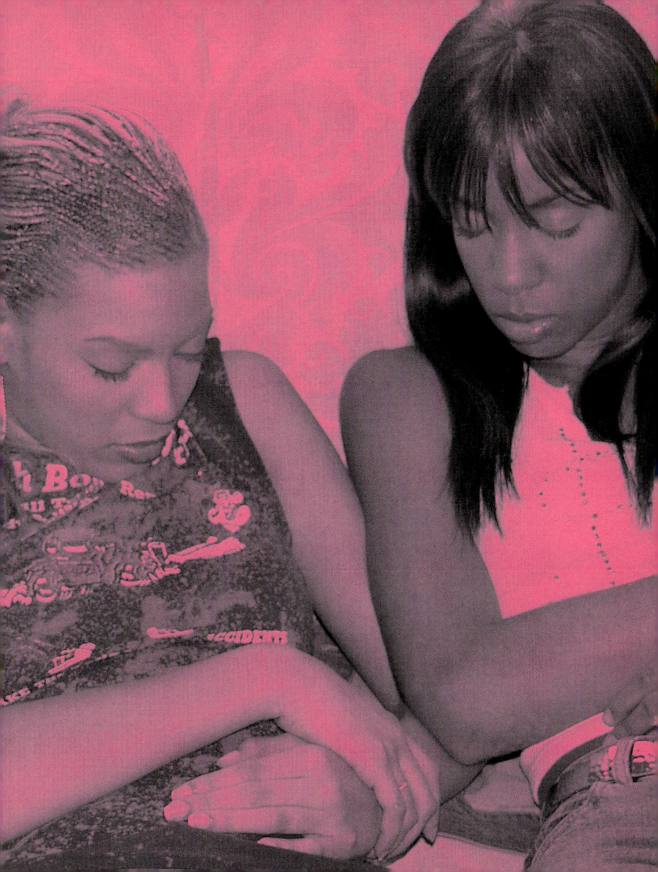

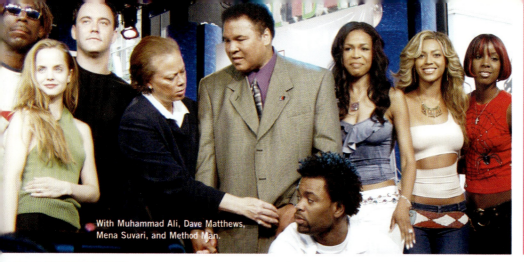

With Muhammad Ali, Dave Matthews, Mena Suvari, and Method Man.

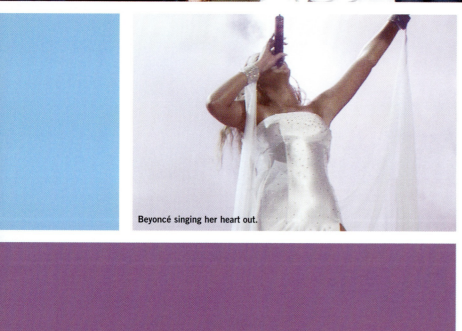

Beyoncé singing her heart out.

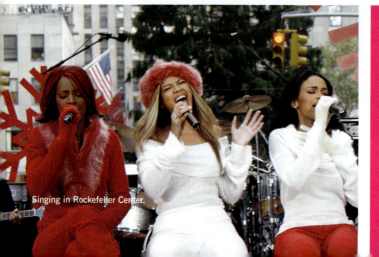

Singing in Rockefeller Center.

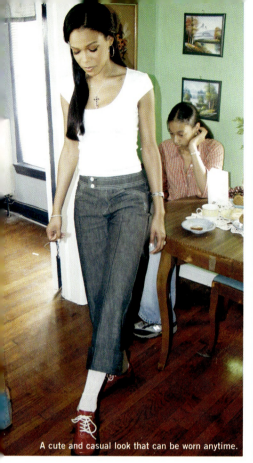
A cute and casual look that can be worn anytime.

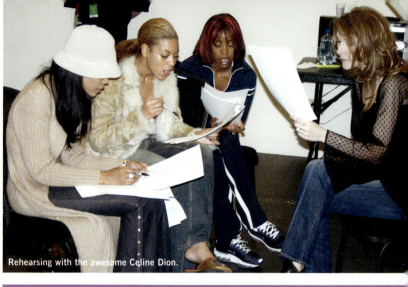
Rehearsing with the awesome Celine Dion.

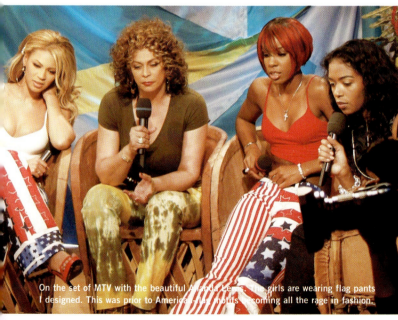
On the set of MTV with the beautiful Ananda Lewis. The girls are wearing flag pants I designed. This was prior to America-flag motifs becoming all the rage in fashion.

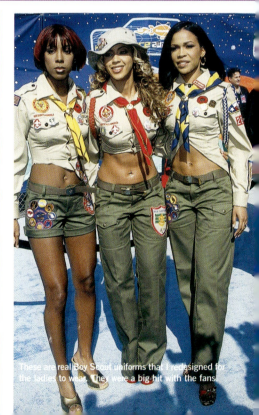
These are real Boy Scout uniforms that I redesigned for the ladies to wear. They were a big hit with the fans.

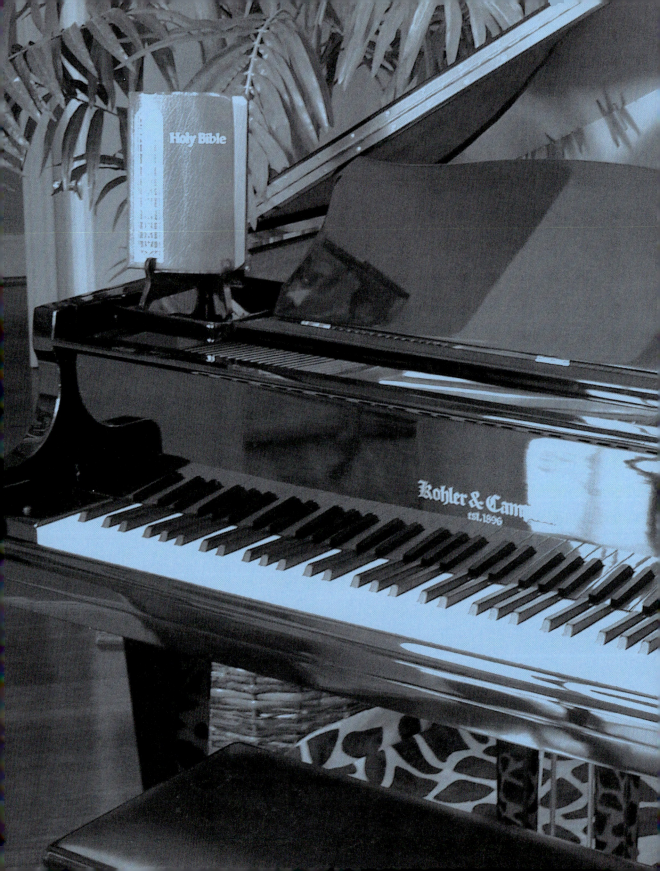

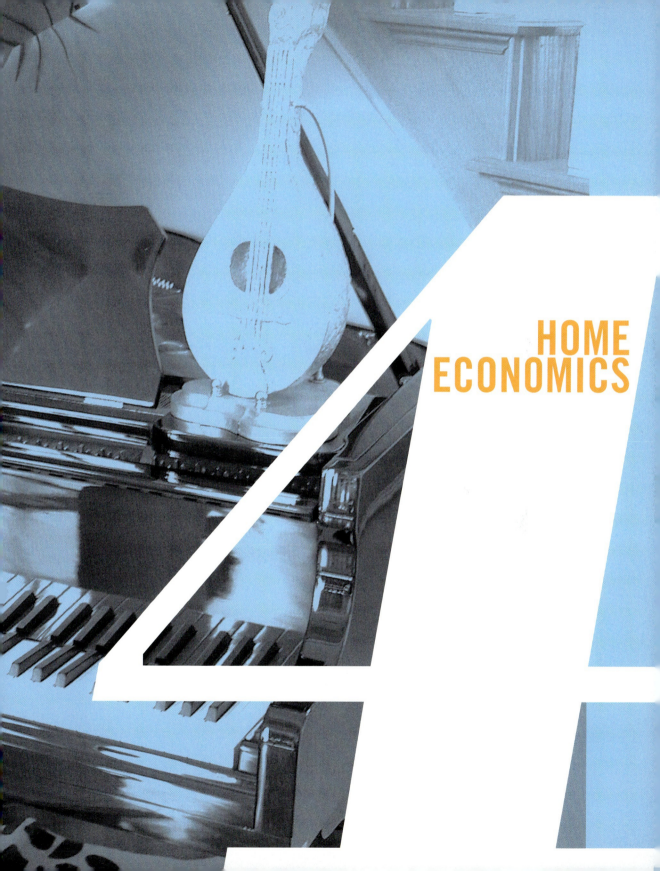

4 HOME ECONOMICS

AS A DECORATOR, I'M COST-CONSCIOUS. I WANT THE BEST VALUE FOR MY DOLLAR. I THINK THAT EVEN IF YOU HAVE MONEY, YOU SHOULDN'T SPEND TOO MUCH FOR THINGS that you can create yourself, especially if it's something that can be done easily and cheaply and doesn't require a lot of time. I like DIY (do-it-yourself) projects because they can give you a sense of artistic satisfaction as well as adding something functional to your home. Besides, instead of just going out and buying everything, I like to add a personal touch. Even with artwork, I'll customize it and give it my own take. In my hair salon, I have a mass-produced print of a painting that I had picked up at a local furniture store and added my own paint to. Now it's a customized one-of-a-kind original. As with my clothes, I never follow rules with decorating. I think your home, apartment, or room should reflect your personal style.

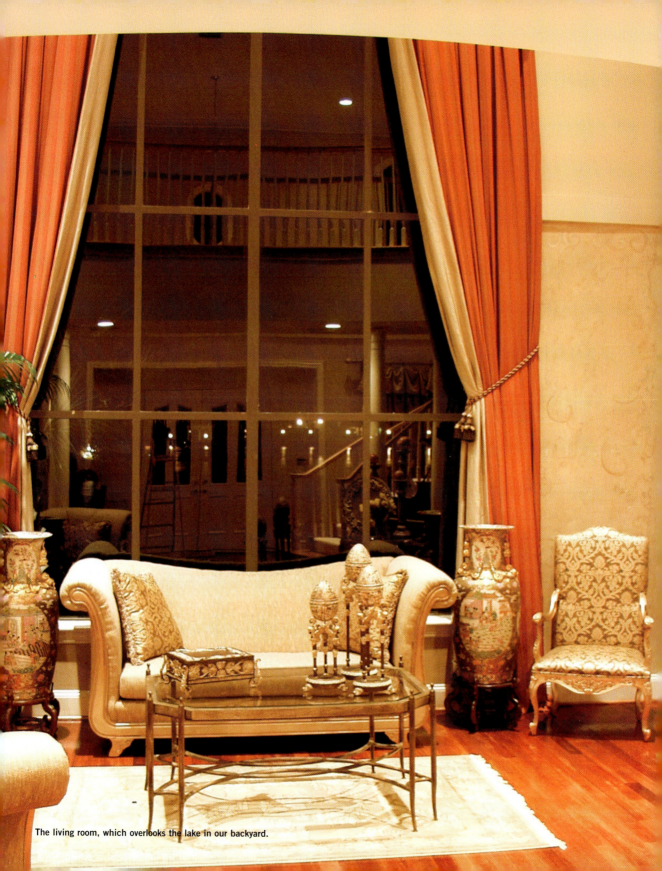
The living room, which overlooks the lake in our backyard.

OUR HOME IS TRULY A GATHERING PLACE FOR THE ENTIRE DESTINY'S CHILD FAMILY. WE'RE NOT HERE VERY OFTEN, BUT WHEN WE ARE IT'S A TREAT FOR EVERYONE TO BE ABLE TO SLEEP IN THEIR OWN BED. KELLY HAS LIVED WITH US SINCE THE GIRLS WERE FIRST STARTING OUT, BECAUSE HER MOM'S WORK SCHEDULE DIDN'T ALLOW HER TO DROP KELLY OFF AND PICK HER UP FROM REHEARSALS. SO WE INVITED HER TO STAY, AND SHE'S LIVED WITH US FOR SEVERAL YEARS NOW. SHE'S A WELCOME ADDITION TO OUR FAMILY, AND WHEN RECENTLY SHE BOUGHT HER OWN HOME IN HOUSTON, I GOT REALLY SAD. BUT I'M SO HAPPY FOR HER AND HAD A BALL HELPING HER DECORATE IT. IT'S A BEAUTIFUL HOME—SIX BEDROOMS IN A GATED COMMUNITY.

Michelle doesn't live at our house, but she has an apartment nearby, which I helped her decorate. She also stays with her parents when she goes home to Rockford, Illinois. When you're on the road as much as DC is, the time you spend at home becomes magical. That's why I really made it a priority to decorate our house (especially Beyoncé's and Kelly's rooms), Beyoncé's apartment in L.A., the house Kelly recently bought, and Michelle's apartment with their personality and individuality in mind.

"our home is truly a gathering place for the entire destiny's child family"

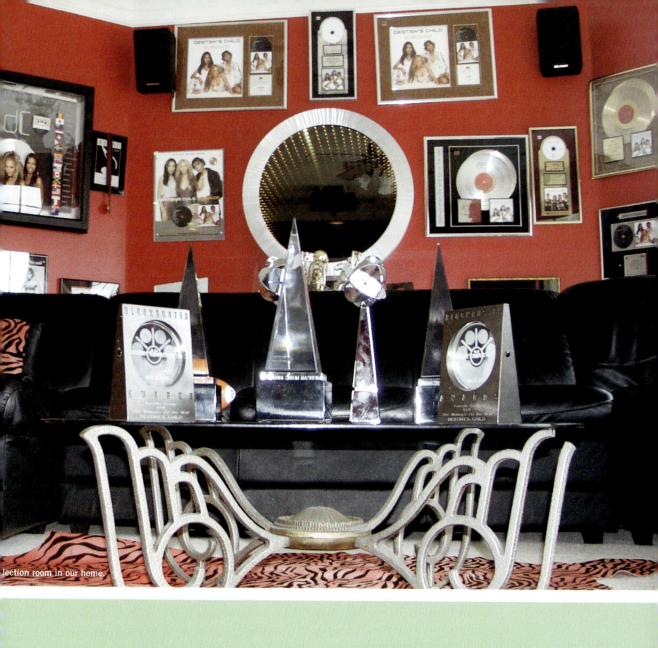

...lection room in our home.

THE SANCTUARY

I'VE ALWAYS BELIEVED THAT THE BEDROOM IS THE MOST IMPORTANT ROOM TO DECORATE. IT'S YOUR SANCTUARY AND IT'S THE PLACE YOU CAN GO AND CLOSE THE DOOR ON THE WORLD AND BE ALONE WITH YOUR THOUGHTS. SO I THINK THE WAY IT'S DECORATED SHOULD REALLY REFLECT YOUR PERSONALITY AND MAKE YOU FEEL RELAXED AND CONTENT. DIFFERENT PEOPLE HAVE DIFFERENT THINGS THAT MAKE THEM FEEL AT EASE. BECAUSE I HAVE A HECTIC LIFE, I LIKE MY BEDROOM TO BE CALM AND PEACEFUL AND SOOTHING, SO I HAVE DIFFERENT SHADES OF BEIGE IN THERE. WITH BEYONCÉ, KELLY, AND MICHELLE, IT'S A WHOLE DIFFERENT STORY.

Beyoncé's room has many colors and is decorated with a strong theme that I call "high drama." Her room is like a fairy tale, which is great for her because it's also her creative space. She writes as she sits on the pillows next to the window that overlooks the lake. She has written most of Destiny's Child's songs in this room, so clearly the combination of bold colors and proximity to the water suits her creativity.

Beyoncé's bedroom is the realization of a longtime dream of hers. Ever since she was a little girl, she always said that whenever she got money she wanted to make her room look like a genie bottle. She got the idea from the TV show *I Dream of Jeannie*. The main character on the show was a woman genie that lived in a bottle. Beyoncé thought it was so pretty with all the colors and pillows. So when Destiny's Child made a video for one of their earlier songs called "With Me" and it had a montage where they were in a genie bottle, I saved the floor pillows that were created for the shoot.

Her bed is the same type of bed that was in the film *The Devil's Advocate* starring Keanu Reeves and Al Pacino. Some time after we saw the movie, we saw a replica of the bed in a furniture store, and Beyoncé had to have it. Once we had the bed, I called a decorative painter over to paint clouds on the ceiling. Then Beyoncé told her about how much she wanted a genie theme, and showed her some fabrics and the pillows we planned on using, and the woman painted the walls to match. I designed the bedspread, which is made out of saris, and when we had it on the bed, Beyoncé decided to hang sari material from the ceiling. The overall look of the room is very dramatic. Even her adjoining bathroom looks like a fairy tale. She has a customized porcelain sink that is painted with a fairy-tale motif—fairies fly around the words to different "Once upon a time" tales.

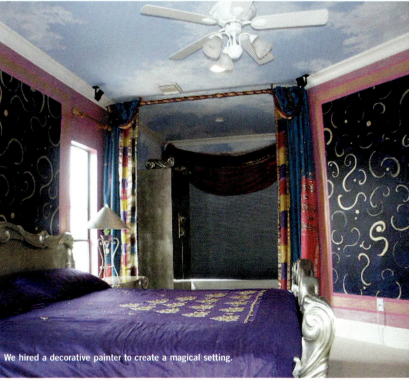
We hired a decorative painter to create a magical setting.

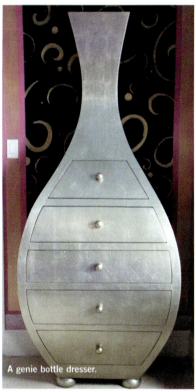
A genie bottle dresser.

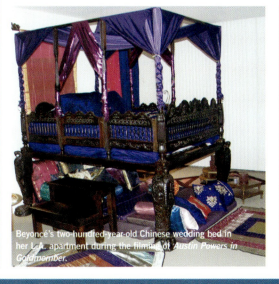
Beyoncé's two-hundred-year-old Chinese wedding bed in her L.A. apartment during the filming of *Austin Powers in Goldmember*.

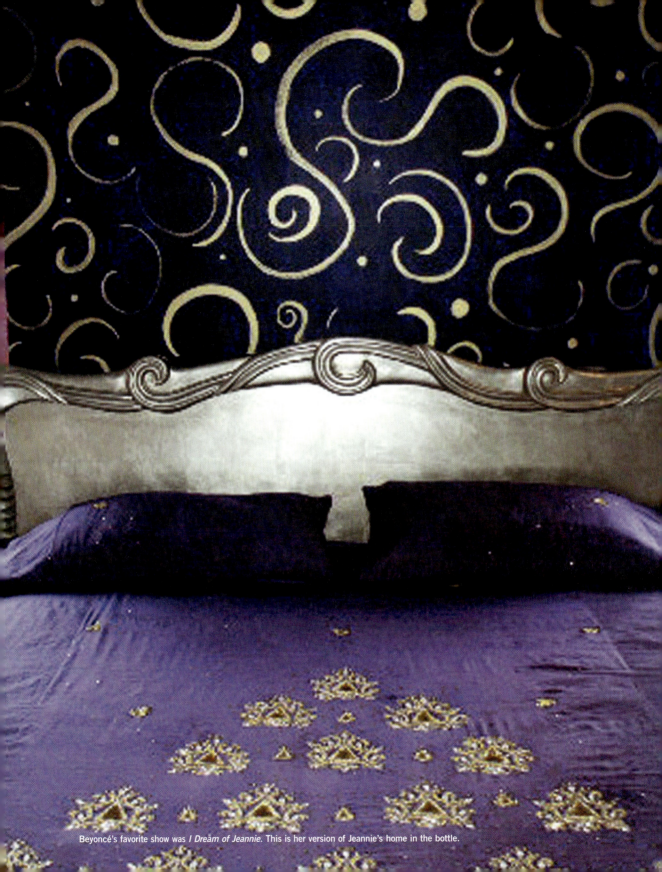

Beyoncé's favorite show was *I Dream of Jeannie*. This is her version of Jeannie's home in the bottle.

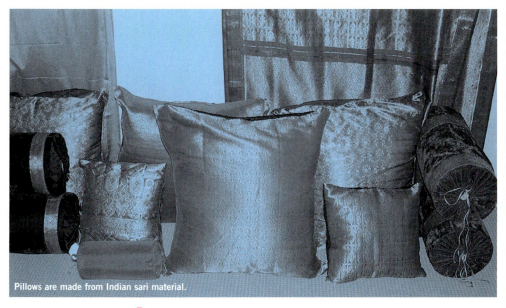
Pillows are made from Indian sari material.

BEYONCÉ'S PILLOWS

1. FIND MATERIAL THAT YOU LIKE AND THAT MATCHES THE LOOK OF THE ROOM. YOU CAN USE BOLD COLORS, ANIMAL PRINTS, FAKE FURS, SATINY MATERIAL—ANYTHING.

2. CUT TWO PIECES OF MATERIAL THE SAME SIZE. THE SIZE OF THE MATERIAL WILL REFLECT THE SIZE OF THE PILLOWS.

3. SEW THEM TOGETHER INSIDE OUT ON THREE SIDES. (YOU CAN SEW BY HAND OR WITH A MACHINE.)

4. TURN THE FABRIC RIGHT SIDE OUT.

5. STUFF WITH FOAM AND SEW THE FOURTH SIDE CLOSED. (IF YOU WANT TO GET FANCY, YOU CAN SEW A ZIPPER ON THE FOURTH SIDE INSTEAD OF SEWING IT CLOSED. THAT WAY YOU CAN CHANGE THE STUFFING WHENEVER YOU WANT.)

I've always thought of Kelly as a princess, so I wanted **Kelly's bedroom** to reflect that. Her room is like a queen's chamber. I used purple and gold to decorate it, because they are rich, opulent colors. She had always wanted a canopy bed, so I found a royal-looking gold one. Next, we needed to find bedding. We looked at a comforter Kelly liked that was premade and cost about two thousand dollars, which didn't include pillows or curtains. Kelly has three extra-large windows in her room, so we wouldn't have been able to buy curtains long enough to fit them. Customizing became a necessity.

She and I went to an interior-decorating store that has fabric at discount prices. We found the same material there that I had seen in a retail fabric store, only it was half the price. There are many high-quality discount fabric stores near our home in Houston. I like going to them because I get really good prices, and the material is the same as regular retail fabric but costs less. You have to look and choose carefully because the fabric may have some kind of little flaw in it, but more often than not, it's simply discounted because it was overstocked or from a past season.

It took a little talking for Kelly to get into purple. At first, she wasn't sure if she would like having a purple room, but when she saw how nice the fabric looked with gold, she was excited about it. Once I saw the fabric we liked, I had visions of how the coordinating fabrics and the design for her comforter and matching curtains should look.

When creating a comforter, I always try to use two different fabrics so that it can be reversible. So on one side of her comforter is a purple and gold zigzag pattern and on the other a purple and gold diamond pattern. The curtain and swags match both materials, and I designed all the pillows to match. The woman who did the sewing is wonderful. I asked her to put three plies of the stuffing material in the comforter so it's heavy, and she was able to sew it easily. By having everything made, I saved several thousand dollars.

"i've always thought of kelly as a princess"

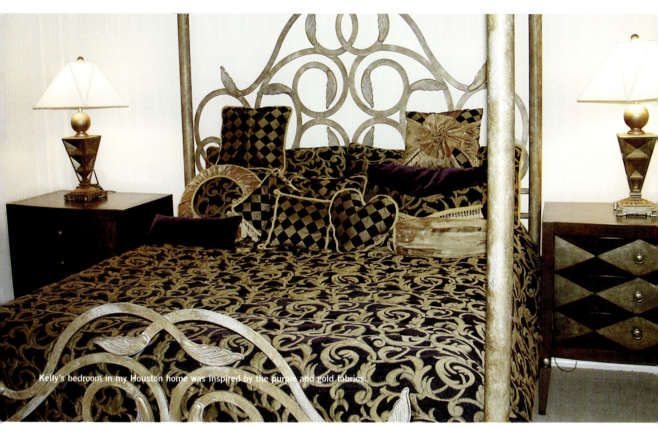

Kelly's bedroom in my Houston home was inspired by the purple and gold fabrics.

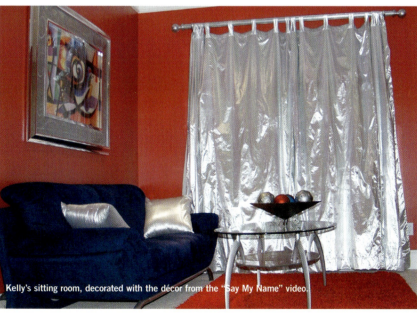

Kelly's sitting room, decorated with the décor from the "Say My Name" video.

HOME ECONOMICS | 169

KELLY'S CUSTOMIZED DUVET

IF YOU WANT TO ADD SOMETHING NEW TO YOUR BEDROOM BUT DON'T HAVE THE MONEY TO BUY A NEW COMFORTER, YOU CAN SEW A DUVET COVER TO PUT OVER YOUR CURRENT BEDDING. IT'S INEXPENSIVE AND EASY TO MAKE. IT'S A VERY SIMILAR METHOD TO MAKING FLOOR PILLOWS. (REFERENCE THE CHART BELOW FOR SIZING INFO.)

1. MEASURE YOUR COMFORTER OR READ THE DIMENSIONS FROM THE ORIGINAL PACKAGING (IF YOU STILL HAVE IT).

2. FIND A FABRIC THAT YOU LIKE. (EXPERIMENT WITH TEXTURES AND MATERIALS FOR FUN. YOU CAN USE ANYTHING FROM FAUX FUR TO VELVET.)

3. CUT TWO IDENTICAL PIECES OF THE MATERIAL FOUR INCHES WIDER THAN YOUR COMFORTER ON ALL SIDES.

4. SEW THREE SIDES OF THE FABRIC TOGETHER WITH THE WRONG SIDES FACING IN.

5. TURN THE SEWN PIECES RIGHT SIDE OUT.

6. FILL THIS WITH YOUR COMFORTER. (IF THE COVER IS A LITTLE LARGE, YOU CAN SECURE THE COMFORTER TO THE INSIDE CORNERS USING SAFETY PINS. THIS KEEPS IT FROM SLIDING AROUND.)

7. YOU CAN EITHER LEAVE THIS SIDE OPEN AND LET IT BE THE SIDE THAT FACES THE TOP WHEN IT'S ON YOUR BED OR YOUR CAN SEW ON A VELCRO STRIP, BUTTONS, OR A ZIPPER TO CLOSE IT UP. (YOU DON'T WANT TO SEW IT, THOUGH, BECAUSE YOU'LL WANT TO BE ABLE TO TAKE YOUR COMFORTER OUT WHEN IT'S TIME TO WASH IT.)

SIZING CHARTS

MATTRESSES

TWIN: 39 × 75 INCHES

FULL/DOUBLE: 54 × 75 INCHES

QUEEN: 60 × 80 INCHES

KING: 78 × 80 INCHES

CALIFORNIA KING: 72 × 82 INCHES

SHEETS

TWIN FLAT: 66 × 96 INCHES

TWIN FITTED: 39 × 75 INCHES

DOUBLE FLAT: 81 × 96 INCHES

DOUBLE FITTED: 54 × 75 INCHES

QUEEN FLAT: 90 × 102 INCHES

QUEEN FITTED: 60 × 80 INCHES

KING FLAT: 100 × 102 INCHES

KING FITTED: 78 × 80 INCHES

CALIFORNIA KING FLAT: 102 × 110 INCHES

CALIFORNIA KING FITTED: 72 × 82 INCHES

A PILLOWCASE SHOULD BE FOUR INCHES LONGER THAN THE PILLOW AND TWO INCHES GREATER IN CIRCUMFERENCE.

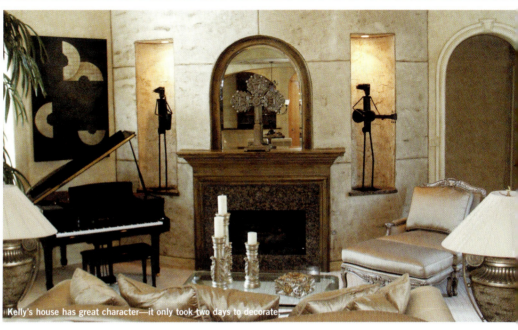
Kelly's house has great character—it only took two days to decorate.

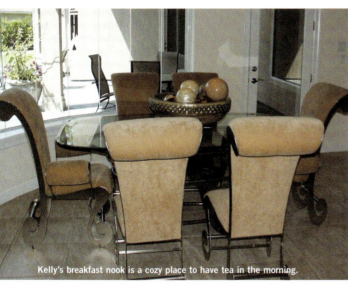
Kelly's breakfast nook is a cozy place to have tea in the morning.

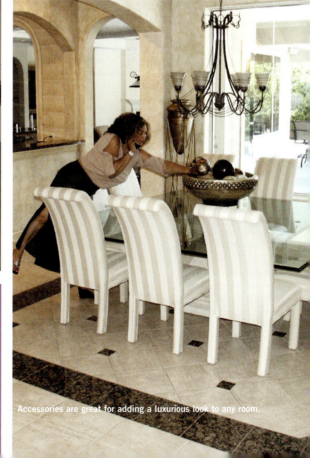
Accessories are great for adding a luxurious look to any room.

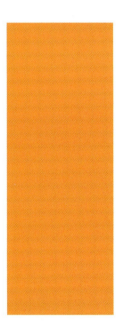

"I used red and beige for her bedroom"

When you live in an apartment, you don't have as much space as you do with a house, so it's critical to make the space you do have more lively. In **Michelle's apartment**, I used red and beige for her bedroom. I felt a red accent would enliven the room and give her a boost of energy, which is important when you live alone. For her living room she selected beautiful off-white leather furniture, so I had one of her walls painted a burnt orange to match the leather Versace throw pillows on her couch. Every room in her place is filled with plants and great vivid accessories.

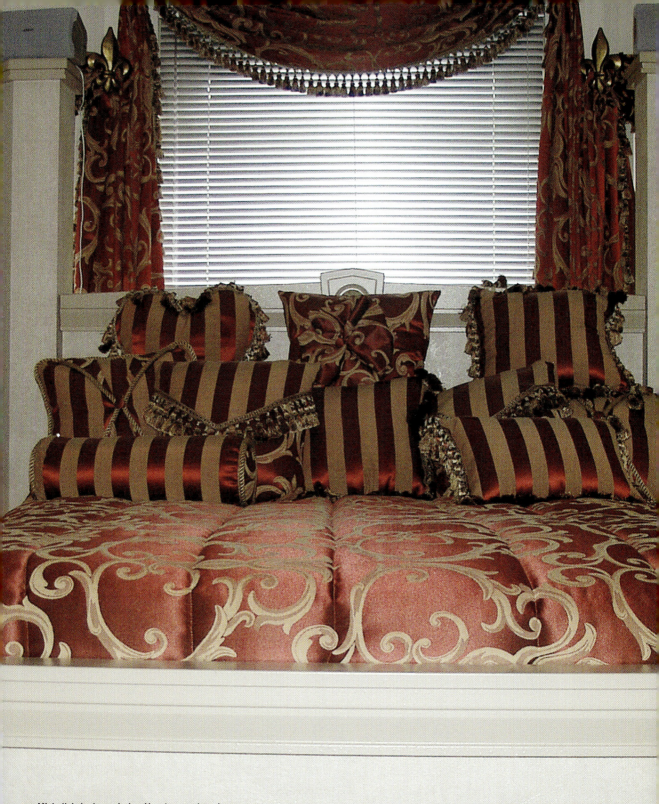
Michelle's bedroom in her Houston apartment.

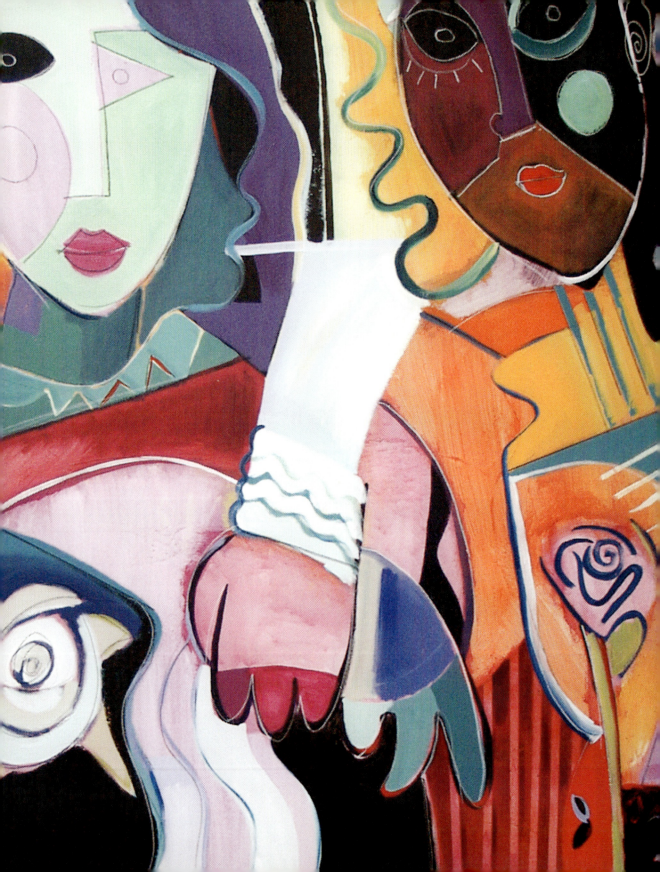

BUDGET DECORATING

My policy on decorating is that first you need to figure out what you have in terms of a budget. I remember my very first apartment—I had *no* budget. However, when I was done decorating everybody loved it. It was a great place. I didn't have any money back then, so I had to be really resourceful. I found an old wicker sofa and matching chair at a garage sale. I got them both for fifty dollars. I had my dad add wood braces to the legs for extra support because the chair and sofa were old and rickety. Next, I painted the wicker a bright yellow. I then found some orange, yellow, and black Oriental fabric that was really inexpensive, which I first used to recover the cushions and with the leftover pieces made lots of big, beautiful overstuffed pillows. I went to another garage sale and picked up a coffee table for only a few dollars. I painted the walls behind the couch orange to tie the look together. Sometimes the craziest things work if you can manage to find even one way to pull the look together. My apartment was the cutest thing, and I was so proud because it was mine. I'd done it myself, and I still had money left to eat. I had spent less than five hundred dollars furnishing my entire apartment.

The key to decorating when you're on a budget is not to fall into the trap that most people do. I see it all the time—people have a fabulous sofa and the rest of the room is empty. You get much more bang for your buck if you buy an inexpensive sofa and leave money to spend on accessories. Throw pillows and paintings are relatively cheap, and you can really personalize your living area with them. They reflect your personality and style.

You can find great accessories at discount stores like T.J. Maxx, Ross, Burlington Coat Factory, and Marshalls. In fact, all the little throw pillows on the couch in my salon I got at stores like those for no more than fifteen dollars apiece. Spray paint is another cheap way to decorate. I'll spray-paint anything in a minute. For Beyoncé's apartment in Los Angeles, I bought a beautiful side table and wanted to put it against a wall in the entry hall and hang a mirror over it. Mirrors can get really pricey, and I didn't want to invest in a big expensive mirror for that apartment because she was only going to live there for six months while filming *Austin Powers in Goldmember*. So I found a mirror I loved at Home Depot, which was perfect size-wise and not that expensive. The only thing wrong with it was that it had a gold-colored frame, and the table that I wanted it to hang over was a silver-leaf (silver over gold) pattern. So I went to the hardware store, got silver glaze, and glazed the gold frame. Then I took a towel and wiped some of the silver paint off so that the gold showed through to match the silver-leaf table. It looks beautiful, and Beyoncé loves it.

My favorite painting.

Fabric Fantasies

Fabric can be your best friend when you're looking to make a dramatic decorating statement without spending a lot of money. It can be used to cover old furniture—like a table, for instance. It's much more economical than purchasing a new one, especially if the only thing wrong with it is cosmetic. Or you can follow Beyoncé's lead and get long, dramatic lengths of fabric and loop them across the ceiling and over your bed and windows. When selecting fabric bear two things in mind: One, make sure the fabric you choose has enough weight and visual drama to achieve the look you want before you commit to it. Light, gauzy fabric is great to drape from ceilings. My advice is to take lots of samples from the fabric store and play around with them until you find the fabric that's just right for the effect you want, so you don't waste money on mistakes. Two, if you are planning to upholster a piece of furniture and are looking for fabric, go to auction houses for really luxe fabrics at good prices, flea markets for cool vintage fabric finds, and fabric discounters who deal in overstocked merchandise from a multitude of fabric stores and have a wide range of contemporary fabrics in a variety of colors and materials. Don't buy it from the upholsterer—you usually won't get as good a price.

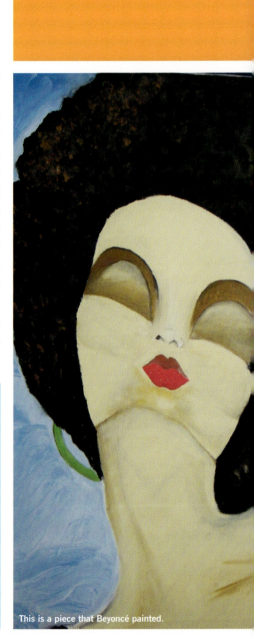

This is a piece that Beyoncé painted.

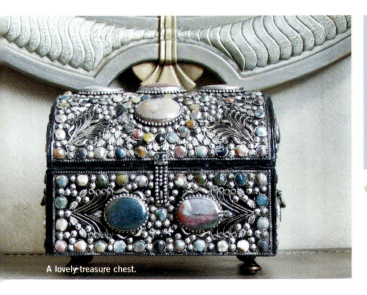
A lovely treasure chest.

"find pieces that speak to you in some way and collect those"

Art-y-facts

The best way to give a room a finished look is to adorn your walls with art. Whenever I mention using art to decorate, people instantly become stressed and say, "But I don't know anything about art." I tell them to calm down and to not be intimidated. Art can be shrouded in mystery, but it's really not that complicated to pull off. The key to collecting art is not to get bogged down with rules about the proper way to display or buy it. Just find pieces that speak to you in some way and collect those. Also check out the art departments at local universities. I've bought some beautiful art from students who I know will be famous one day, but are starving artists right now.

If you immerse yourself in the process of looking at art for one day a week, by the end of a month, you'll have a good sense of what you like and don't like style-wise. Go to very small galleries run by local artists; there you can negotiate a good price because it's their art and they run the gallery. Collect art that isn't "trendy" at the moment. You'll get a better price, and you may even become a trendsetter. If you have offbeat taste, hit secondhand stores and pick up secondhand art that you like. Religious art and strange little portraits from unknown artists can be found at places like this, especially if you don't like the mass-produced prints of famous paintings that are sold in many stores. Most important, remember to start small. You don't have to get a huge, fancy piece of art to make a statement. You can buy groupings of smaller prints or paintings. Then if you move, transporting the art won't be such a production.

OFFICE STYLE

YOUR OFFICE IS WHEREVER YOU SPEND MOST OF YOUR TIME WORKING. IT DOESN'T MATTER IF IT'S A CUBICLE IN A FORTUNE 500 COMPANY, THE PLUSH CORNER OFFICE IN A SWANK BUILDING IN THE MIDDLE OF YOUR TOWN'S BUSINESS DISTRICT, OR THE ALCOVE UNDERNEATH THE STAIRS IN YOUR HOUSE, YOUR OFFICE IS WHERE YOU HANDLE YOUR PROFESSIONAL COMMUNICATION WITH THE OUTSIDE WORLD. NO MATTER WHERE IT IS OR WHAT SIZE IT IS, IT'S IMPORTANT THAT YOUR OFFICE MOTIVATES, INSPIRES, AND REFLECTS WHO YOU ARE AND WHAT YOU'RE TRYING TO ACCOMPLISH WITH YOUR CAREER.

My husband is the founder and CEO of Music World Entertainment, an artist-management company and record label. His clients include Destiny's Child and all three members as solo artists, our daughter Solange, the rapper Nas, a group from Sweden called Play, a boy group called Signature, and two solo female singers, Chelsea Smith and Devin. As you can imagine, Mathew spends a lot of time in his office and he's definitely one of those people who works nonstop. There's no such thing as an eight-hour workday for him, so I wanted to create an atmosphere that empowered him. We're both fans of African art, so in his office I incorporated lots of art and artifacts like spears, drums, and masks. Basically, when you think about it, the job of a music executive is to be a warrior, to fight to get the artists' music and image out there. So the theme here works well.

Shortly after I decorated Mathew's office, I received a phone call from a man who was a serious art collector near our home in Houston. He said, "Mrs. Knowles, I hear you're into African art and that you have some exquisite pieces." Before I could even say anything, he continued talking, and it turned out that his partner, who was part of an investment group with Mathew, had seen the office and reported back to his friend how we were into collecting African art. He was very excited, said he had museum-quality pieces, and was interested in getting together to look at some pieces I had. I had to laugh and tell him most of the pieces I had came from Marshalls, a discount store that carries home goods and clothing. They were actual African carvings, but these were not by any means one-of-a-kind originals. In fact, they were all discounted and in the sale bin. It just goes to show that you don't have to spend a fortune to make a room look like you did.

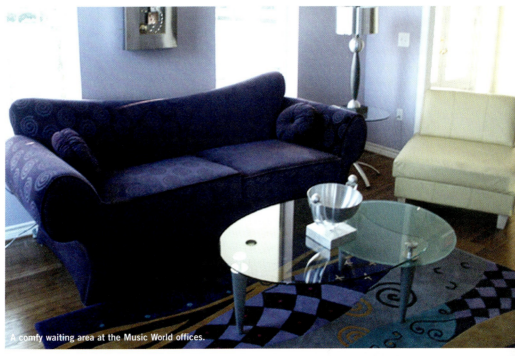
A comfy waiting area at the Music World offices.

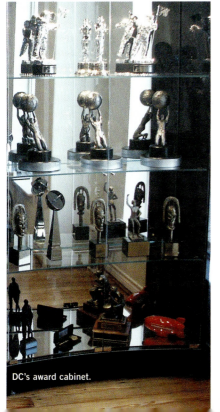
DC's award cabinet.

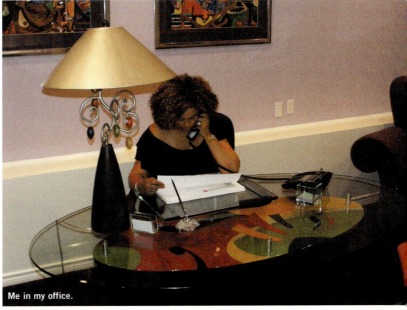
Me in my office.

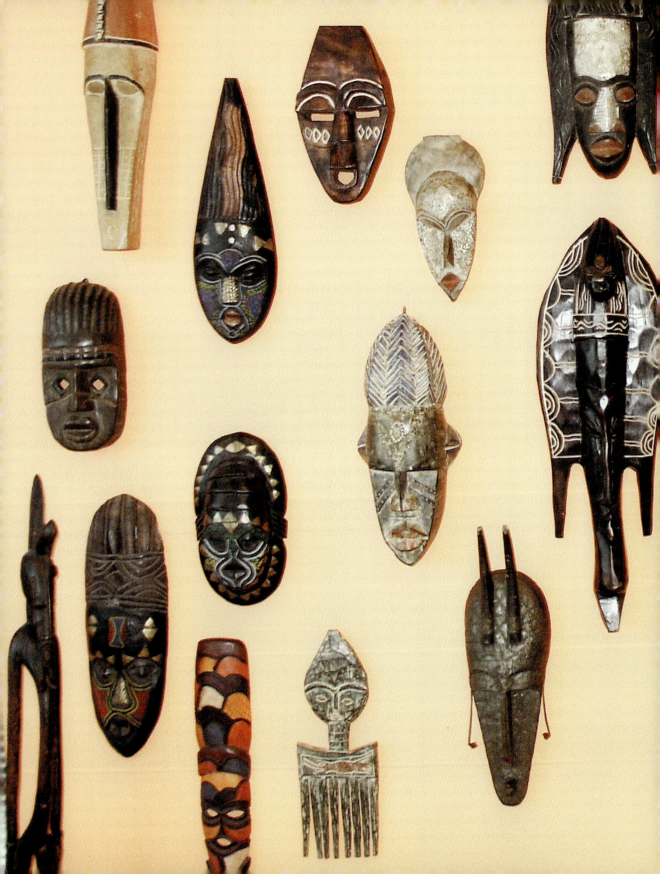

ETHNIC DECORATING ON A BUDGET

When you're working with a stong ethnic theme, like African, Indian, or Middle Eastern, it's important to be consistent. I've seen too many people who start off with good intentions for a room and somewhere in the middle of the process they veer off in a whole other direction. For instance, if you have decided to create an Asian-inspired theme in your home, I recommend figuring out your color scheme next. Let's say your main color is going to be red, with accent colors of white and black. If you stick to those colors when shopping for accessories and furnishings you'll be fine. It's when people don't stay focused that they get into trouble theme-wise and budget-wise. If you start buying things that look cute without giving any thought to your original vision, you'll have a bunch of great stuff when you get home but none of it will go together or carry out the theme you originally had in mind. To combat impulse buying make a list of what you're looking for before you leave the house and stick to it. If you need a lamp, a chair, and a painting buy those first. Then if you have money left over, you can get the cute little picture frame that you came across when looking for a lamp.

When it comes time to accessorize with arts and crafts for the theme you've selected, remember to keep the personality of the furniture in tune with the personality of the accessories. For example, in Mathew's office, the masks, drums, and spears make bold statements, so I used substantial and strong wood furniture to go along with it. The overall effect of the room would not have been as striking if I'd used delicate office furniture in soft colors.

Another thing to keep in mind is that ethnic artifacts, regardless of how much you paid for them, need to be displayed properly. They look best with plenty of space around them. That way each piece stands on it own, and your arrangement doesn't look cluttered.

TIPS FOR DECORATING WITH AN AFRICAN FLAIR

- Choose chunky, clean-edged designs for furniture in dark, tropical woods, black lacquer, or blond woods.

- The pieces you choose don't have to be authentically African; just make sure that they are balanced and displayed in an uncluttered manner in the room.

- Faux animal skins work well in this motif. Just don't go overboard—you don't want too many hides lying around, or it starts to look tacky.

- Carved wooden bowls or busts, drums, and spears, and figures of birds, and other animals add drama to the room.

- Cotton or silk Kente cloths can be draped on walls or used as window treatments.

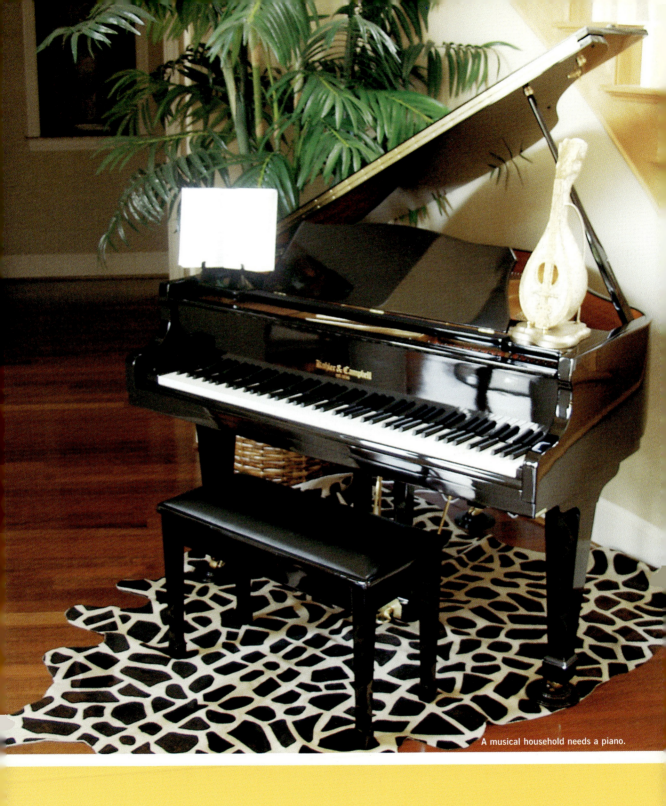

A musical household needs a piano.

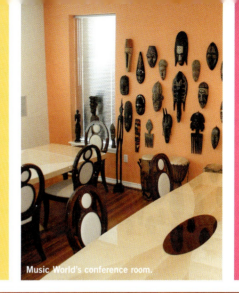

Music World's conference room.

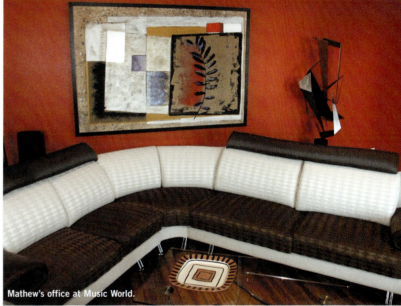

Mathew's office at Music World.

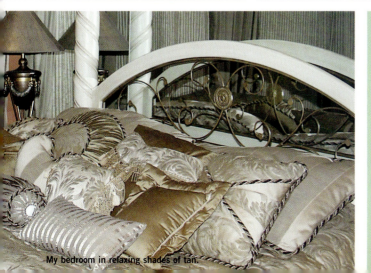

My bedroom in relaxing shades of tan.

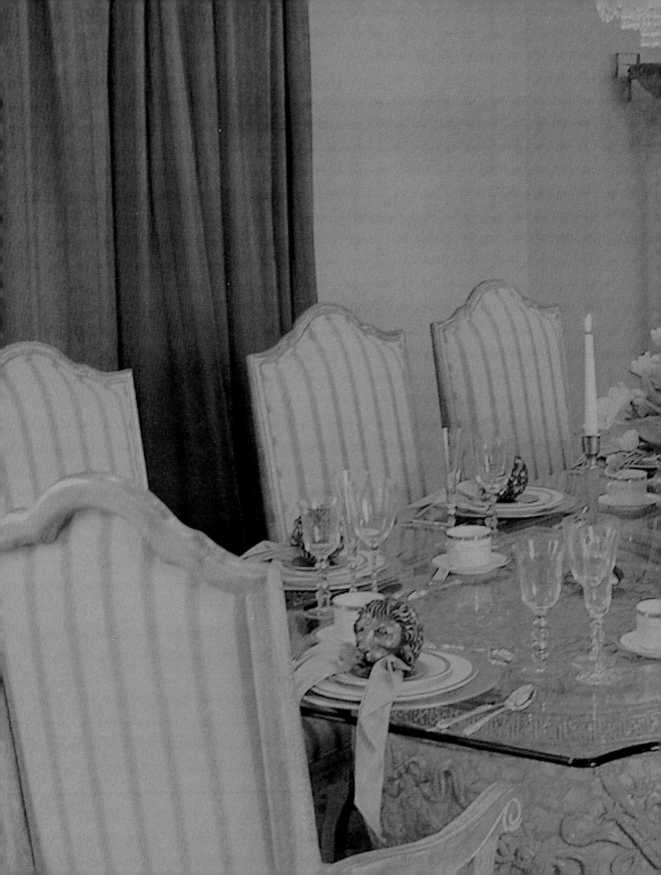

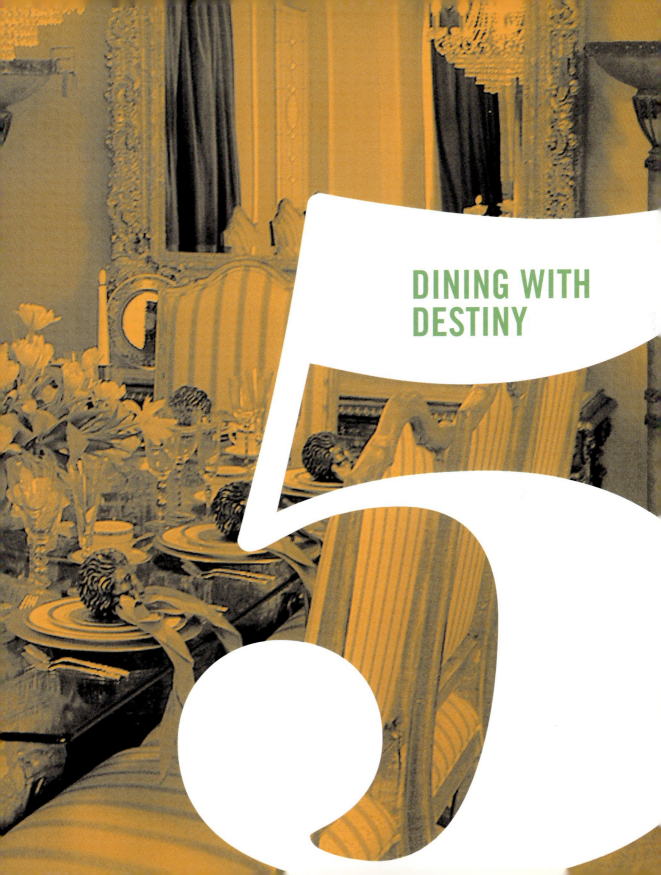

5

DINING WITH DESTINY

I'M VERY INFORMAL WHEN IT COMES TO ENTERTAINING. BEFORE DC TOOK OFF, AND OUR LIVES WERE SOMEWHAT MORE STRUCTURED, I TOOK GREAT PRIDE IN HAVING BIG AND ELABORATE FORMAL DINNERS ON SPECIAL OCCASIONS. NOW THAT WE'RE NOT HOME MUCH, WE PREFER TO HAVE CASUAL, LAID-BACK CELEBRATIONS.

I like an informal atmosphere that's all about family, friends, and good food. The best times are had when you keep it simple. Holiday dinners are low-maintenance, as are everyday celebrations. When we have guests in town, we take them to church and have dinner afterward. Church and dinner every Sunday is a Knowles family tradition.

The kind of cooking I like to do is quick and easy. I used to get frustrated when I'd buy cookbooks and they had long complicated recipes that required me to spend a fortune at the grocery store. That's fine for some people, but when I cook I like to keep it simple. For every holiday I make a big pot of gumbo and serve it buffet style. I lay the food out and everyone gets up and fixes their own plate. Then we sit down at the table, say grace, and eat. Meals are a lot more fun and the food stays hotter when you're not being all formal and passing the plates around. This way you can just dig in and enjoy the food. I have a thing about eating when the food is hot. I'm a real easy-going person—but don't let my food get cold, or you'll see me get very upset.

As for setting the table, I've never used exquisite fine china because I've always had a lot of kids at my house. If they broke something, I wanted to be able to replace it and not have to grieve over it. Even though the kids are now grown, I still buy plates from stores like Ikea. They're inexpensive and practical, and the simple, classic style goes with every occasion. This past Christmas Beyoncé and Kelly bought me the whole collection of Versace tableware. It is beautiful and will be a great heirloom to pass down to my daughters. The retail price on the collection was several thousand dollars, so it isn't really practical for everyday use. I love my Versace dishes, but you don't have to spend a lot of money on your dishes to have an elegant-looking table. I have a set of dishes that cost what one serving dish costs from my Versace set and when I set the table, no one can tell that the all the dishes and silverware in the set cost less than a hundred dollars.

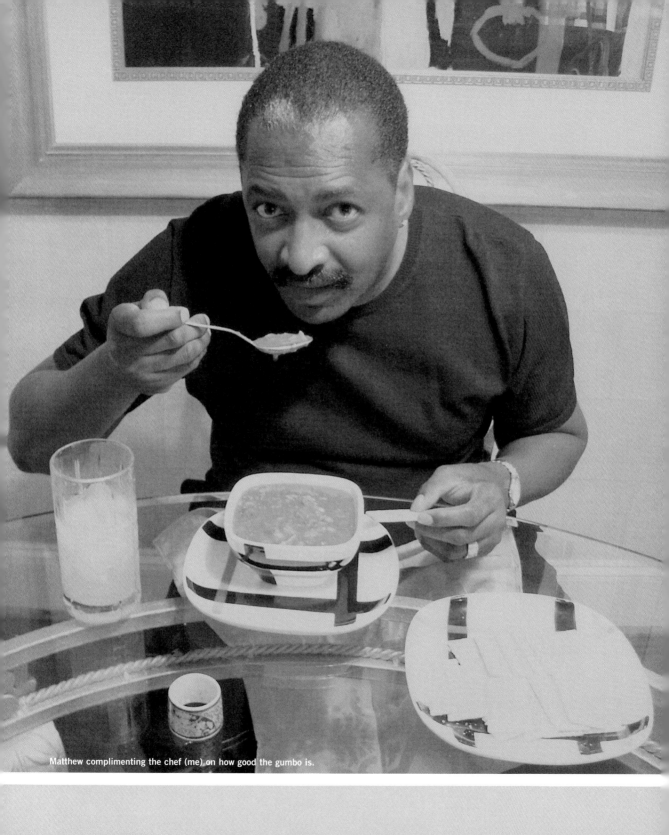
Matthew complimenting the chef (me) on how good the gumbo is.

EXPENSIVE

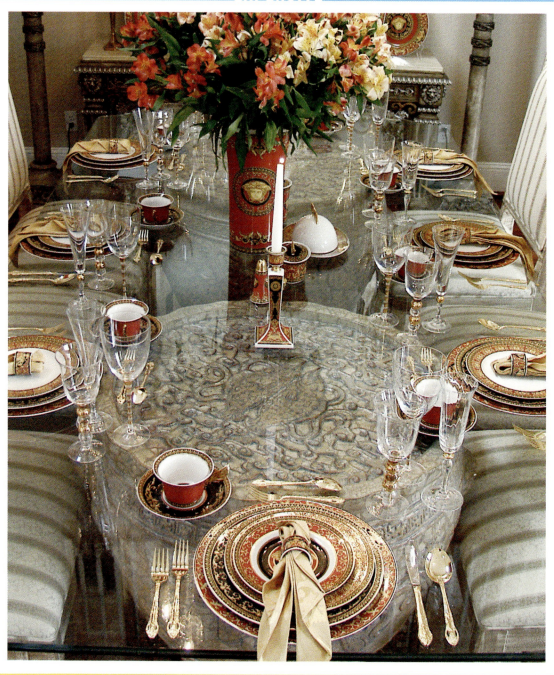

Total cost: $16,000.00
This total doesn't even include the flatware or glassware! I used the same economical glasses and flatware you see in the inexpensive table setting—and you can't tell the difference!

INEXPENSIVE

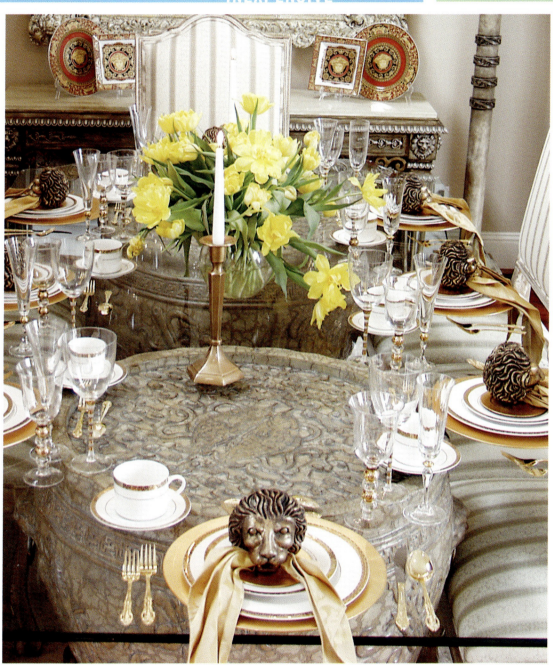

Total Cost: $531.67
Dishes from Bed, Bath & Beyond: $59.99
Glasses from Target: Large 8 @ $5.99 each = $47.92
Medium: 8 @ $4.99 each = $39.92
Small: 8 @ $2.99 each = $23.92
Gold flatware from Target: $50.00 for an 8-piece setting
Lion head napkin holders from Home Depot Expo: 8 @ $20.00 each = $160.00
Napkins from Bed, Bath & Beyond: 8 @ $4.00 each = $32.00
Gold charge plates from Ross: 8 @ $5.00 each = $40.00
Candle holders: 8 @ $5.99 each = $47.92
Gold coasters $6.00 per box
Tulips: $24.00

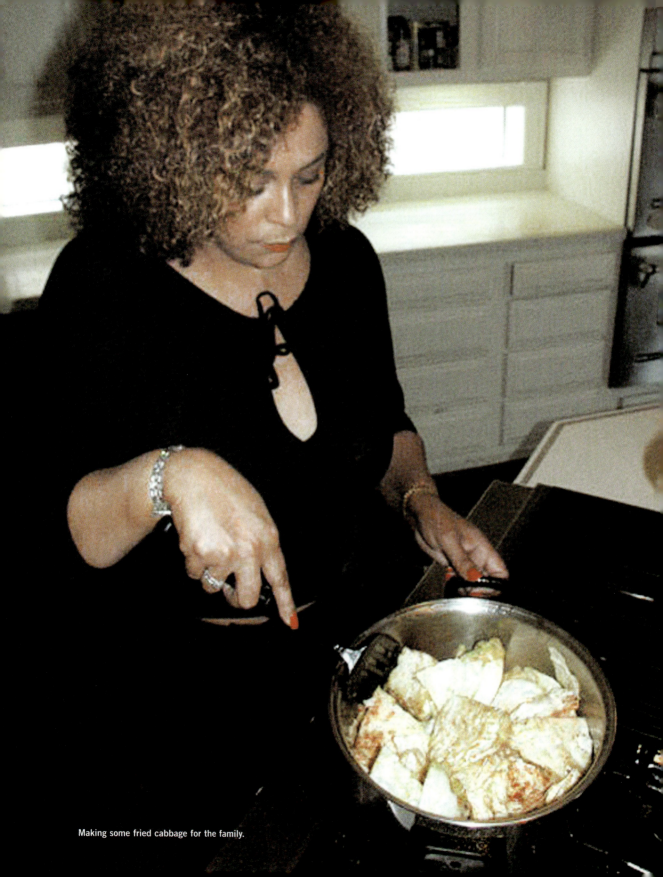
Making some fried cabbage for the family.

HOME COOKING

The way I was raised influenced the way I cook now. My family's tradition growing up was typically Creole. On Christmas Eve we'd go to midnight mass and then come home and each open one gift. Then the next morning we woke up and opened all our gifts. Mathew and I used to do that with the girls, but now the tradition has changed. We get up early on Christmas Day, each read a verse out of the Bible about the birth of Christ, and then open all the gifts. After that, we sing Christmas carols, which may sound really corny, but it's the truth. We hang around in our pajamas all day and usually eat right at noon.

I do the majority of the cooking, but I do get some help. Kelly loves to make banana pudding, and Beyoncé's the official table-setter. She jokes that she makes great ice. She can cook, she just doesn't always choose to anymore. When she was fifteen she used to make dinner every night for the girls in the group because I worked a lot and wasn't always home on time. She cooked steak, Hamburger Helper, Tuna Helper, and that kind of stuff. She'd make salads and feed everyone. Now she really doesn't have the time to cook. Although this past Christmas she did make the yams.

Buffet Style

I've found a buffet is the best way to feed any size group. It's ideal for big family celebrations because it is informal and allows you a great deal of flexibility and ease, which is essential when you're dealing with a diverse mix of meat eaters, vegetarians, family, friends, young children, and adults.

A buffet will work any time of day and for any occasion, from a holiday dinner to a weekend brunch. Just remember to plan a menu that includes food that can be served at room temperature and will hold up well while sitting out on your buffet table.

Buffets can be a messy situation since people help themselves, so cover your buffet table with a tablecloth or something that can take the abuse of spills and protect the table underneath. Make sure to position the serving table for easy access with enough space for people to move around and fill their plates without bumping into anything. For large buffet parties, it's a good idea to have separate tables with different food on each one—entrées like turkey, ham, or fish on one table, side dishes on another, desserts on another. This helps maintain the flow, so if someone is caught up in a web of confusion over trying to decide what to pick next, the person behind can move on and grab another dish. The dining table should be set beforehand with glasses, napkins, and silverware, so the guests can focus on getting their food. Also, chafing dishes are invaluable because they keep food hot for long periods of time. They are worth the investment. You can rent them as well.

The Menu

Gumbo and Cajun turkey are two of my family's favorite dishes. To go with the turkey, I make a cornbread dressing and baked macaroni and cheese—it's very fattening, but good. I also serve greens and yams. Sometimes I'll make fried okra, but that's hard to keep hot so it's not the best buffet food.

Here are some of the recipes that are favorites at my home. I hope they become favorites at yours as well.

Tina's Creole Gumbo

INGREDIENTS

APPROXIMATELY 1 CUP VEGETABLE OIL

2½ CUPS FLOUR

6 ONE-POUND BAGS CUT FROZEN OKRA, DEFROSTED

1 TABLESPOON VINEGAR

3 GALLONS WATER

½ BUNCH CELERY, CHOPPED

3 LARGE BELL PEPPERS (ANY COLOR), CHOPPED

4 YELLOW ONIONS, CHOPPED

3 BUNCHES OF GREEN ONIONS, CHOPPED

1½ CUPS MCCORMICK SEASONING SALT

¼ CUP GARLIC POWDER

¼ CUP ACCENT SEASONING

4 TABLESPOONS CAYENNE PEPPER

4 TABLESPOONS BLACK PEPPER

1 DOZEN MEDIUM-SIZE CRABS, OR 1½ DOZEN SMALL CRABS, CLEANED BUT STILL IN THE SHELL

6 LARGE CHICKEN BREASTS, CUT INTO CHUNKS

15 LARGE CHICKEN DRUMSTICKS

1 16-OUNCE CAN TOMATOES, DICED

6 POUNDS BEEF SAUSAGE, SLICED INTO DISKS

6 POUNDS UNCOOKED MEDIUM-SIZE SHRIMP, PEELED AND DEVEINED

RICE (FOLLOW INSTRUCTIONS ON BOX FOR THE DESIRED AMOUNT)

I USUALLY SERVE GUMBO FOR ALL MY SPECIAL OCCASIONS; IT'S BECOME MY TRADEMARK RECIPE. IN FACT, RAPPER JAY-Z LIKES IT SO MUCH THAT HE'LL FLY TO HOUSTON JUST TO HAVE A BOWL.

THE NICE THING ABOUT GUMBO IS THAT ONCE THE ORIGINAL COOKING PROCESS IS DONE, YOU CAN LET IT SIT ON THE STOVE WITHOUT HEAT AND, THE LONGER IT SITS, THE MORE FLAVOR COMES OUT. GUMBO KEEPS IN THE REFRIGERATOR FOR SEVERAL DAYS AND FREEZES NICELY. NO TWO BATCHES OF GUMBO ARE EVER THE SAME. NO MATTER HOW MANY TIMES I'VE MADE IT, I NEVER CAN DUPLICATE IT EXACTLY.

1. To make the roux: Pour the vegetable oil into a skillet so that the bottom is covered and heat over medium to medium-high heat. Add the flour a little at a time until it's all blended. Add the rest of the oil as needed. Stir constantly until it's browned to a dark fudge consistency. You know you are rockin' the roux when it changes from a peanut-butter shade to a dark chocolate color. This takes about 45 minutes. The key to roux is not to scorch it. If the roux starts to get darker than a peanut-butter color before a half hour has passed, the heat is too high. If that happens, remove the pan from the stove, still stirring, and turn down the heat a little. Let the burner cool down for a while before placing the pan back on the stove. It may take some experimenting before you find the right setting. If you burn the roux it will kill the taste of your gumbo, so you'll have to throw it away, clean the utensils, and start over. *2.* In another skillet, fry the okra. The secret is to cook the okra so that when you add it to your gumbo it isn't slimy and mushy. Cover the bottom of the skillet with about 3 tablespoons of oil and heat over low to medium heat. Add the okra. Then add about a teaspoon of vinegar (this cuts down on the slime) and continue to stir-fry the okra. Whenever you see it getting a little slimy, add a splash of vinegar.

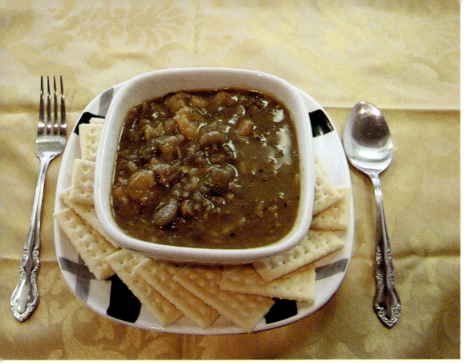

Also add oil to prevent sticking as needed. You don't want to cook it to death, so I'd say no more than 15 minutes' frying time for a whole bag.
3. To make the gumbo: Pour the water into a large gumbo pot and add the celery, bell peppers, onions, green onions, and all the seasonings. You do not want to boil the vegetables. You want to slow-cook them so that the flavor comes out, so set your stove on low to medium heat and leave it there while you add the crabs, chicken, tomatoes, sausage, and cooked okra. Pour in the roux, but stir gently as you add it to make sure that it separates into the water evenly. Taste to check the seasoning. To make it less spicy, add more water, or to make it spicier, add more of the seasonings. Simmer, covered, over low to medium heat for three to four hours or until the meat is nice and tender, and the flavor is rich and robust. There are no shortcuts, so you are going to have to baby-sit that pot until it's ready. Stir it frequently with an extralong spoon that reaches to the bottom of the pot. Add the shrimp a few minutes before the gumbo is served. They will turn pink when done. **4.** Serve over rice.

SERVES 12, WITH LEFTOVERS

Tina's Spicy Cajun Turkey

INGREDIENTS

- 4 TABLESPOONS McCORMICK SEASONING SALT
- 1 TABLESPOON GARLIC POWDER
- 1 TABLESPOON ONION POWDER
- 1 TABLESPOON CAYENNE PEPPER
- 1 TABLESPOON ACCENT SEASONING
- 1 TEN- TO TWELVE-POUND TURKEY
- 2 TABLESPOONS FLOUR

ANOTHER FAMILY FAVORITE IS MY CAJUN TURKEY. I USE AN INJECTION KIT TO SHOOT THE TURKEY FULL OF A SEASONING MIXTURE I MAKE FROM A VARIETY OF SPICES. (YOU CAN FIND INJECTION KITS ONLINE AT SITES LIKE OUTDOORCOOKING.COM OR IN YOUR GROCERY STORE.) FOR ADDED FLAVOR, I PLACE AN ONION AND SOME GARLIC INSIDE THE TURKEY.

I ALSO USE REYNOLDS COOKING BAGS, WHICH CAN BE PICKED UP IN ANY GROCERY STORE. WHEN YOU'RE LEARNING TO COOK, COOKING BAGS ARE YOUR BEST FRIEND. WHEN I WAS FIRST LEARNING, MY MOM SAID, "YOU'RE NOT GETTING THIS RIGHT, SO USE A COOKING BAG." A COOKING BAG CUTS YOUR COOKING TIME IN HALF BECAUSE ALL THE HEAT IS COMPRESSED, AND IT KEEPS IN ALL THE JUICES AND FLAVORS, WHICH IS GREAT FOR BASTING. IT IS THE KEY TO GOOD TASTING MEAT.

To make the injection kit seasoning: **1.** Place 1/2 cup water in a small saucepan and bring to a boil over medium heat. **2.** Add the seasoning salt, garlic powder, onion powder, cayenne pepper, and Accent. **3.** Boil until the mixture becomes a smooth liquid. Turn off the heat.

To prepare the bird: **1.** Defrost the turkey thoroughly if it's frozen. Wash the turkey well. **2.** Fill the turkey injector with the seasoning liquid and inject into the turkey meat. The more places you inject the seasoning, the spicier it will be. I inject it all over the place—after all, I am Creole. If you know there is someone who likes a particular part of the bird and can't take spicy food, then avoid injecting that part. **3.** Put two tablespoons of flour in a cooking bag, then hold the end closed and shake the bag so that the flour coats it. **4.** Place the turkey inside the bag, and then place it in a roasting pan that's big enough to accommodate the bird. **5.** Seal the bag and use a fork to punch about six holes in the top of the bag. Follow the instructions on the bag for cooking time. **6.** When the turkey is done, carefully pour the juice from the bag into a cup. Slice the turkey on a serving platter and pour the juice over the slices. Serve immediately. **SERVES 8**

as we say in louisiana, now that's good eating!

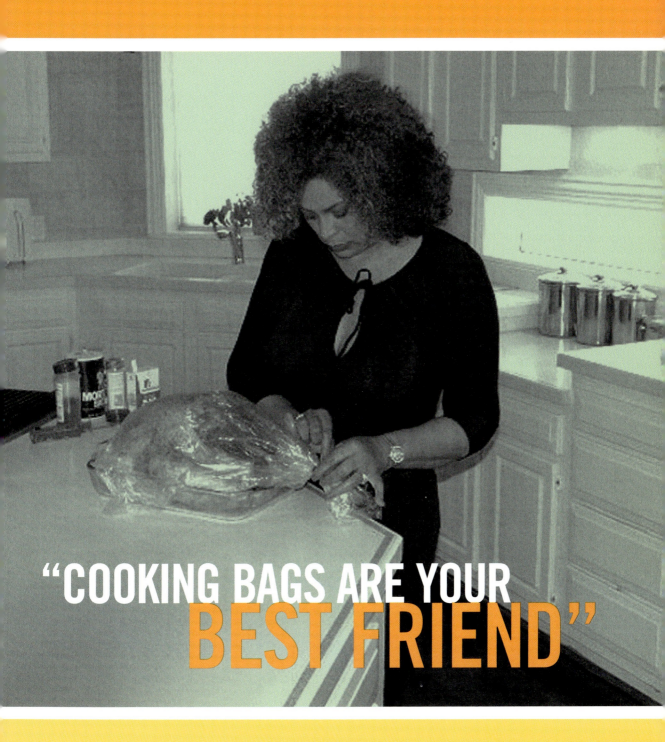

Ten-Minute Cajun Green Bean Stir-fry

INGREDIENTS

4 SLICES PORK BACON (OR 6 SLICES TURKEY BACON)

1 ONION, CHOPPED

1-OUNCE CAN NEW POTATOES, DRAINED

2 1-QUART CANS GREEN BEANS, DRAINED

2 TABLESPOONS MCCORMICK SEASONING SALT

1 TEASPOON BLACK PEPPER

½ TEASPOON CAYENNE PEPPER POWDER

½ TEASPOON GARLIC POWDER

¼ TEASPOON ACCENT SEASONING

BEYONCÉ LOVES THIS! IT'S AN EASY DISH TO PREPARE FOR A BUFFET AND IS GREAT FOR ANY OCCASION. IT GOES REALLY WELL WITH THE CAJUN TURKEY.

1. Heat a wok until it's very hot. Fry the bacon until it starts to curl and turn brown, but don't wait for it to be completely done. *2.* Swirl the wok around a little so that the bacon grease coats the bottom and sides. *3.* Add the onion and cook until it starts to turn clear. *4.* Add the potatoes and the green beans, and cook until they are done to a texture you like, then add all the spices. You can modify the amounts of seasonings or omit some to suit your taste. *5.* Stir-fry until all the vegetables are coated with the seasonings and serve.

SERVES 4 TO 6

Stir-fried Cabbage

THIS DISH IS A FAVORITE OF MICHELLE'S. IT'S SPICY, SO BE CAREFUL!

INGREDIENTS

- PAM COOKING SPRAY
- 1 LARGE HEAD OF GREEN CABBAGE, CHOPPED
- 2 TABLESPOONS MCCORMICK SEASONING SALT
- ½ TEASPOON CAYENNE PEPPER
- 1 TEASPOON BLACK PEPPER
- ½ TEASPOON GARLIC POWDER
- ¼ TEASPOON ACCENT SEASONING

1. Lightly spray your wok with cooking spray and heat the wok to high. 2. Add the cabbage, but keep stirring so that it doesn't stick to the bottom of the wok. Do not add water, since cabbage makes its own water when it's cooked. 3. Add all the seasonings. Stir-fry until you reach your desired texture. I like my cabbage cooked well, while some people like it slightly cooked and still crispy. It's up to you. 4. Just remember, cabbage only takes a minute of hesitation on your part to burn.

SERVES 4 TO 6

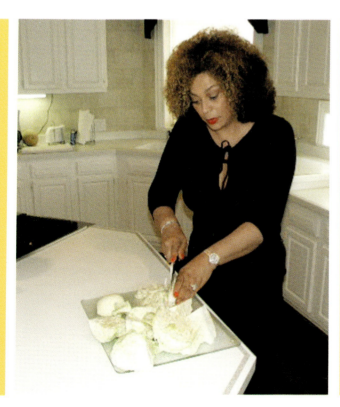
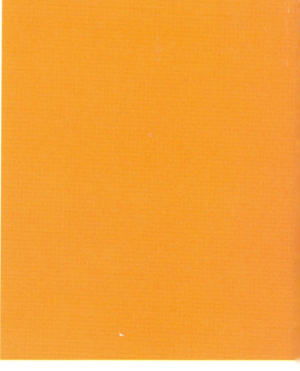

Candied Yams

INGREDIENTS

- 8 LARGE YAMS
- ½ CUP BROWN SUGAR
- 2½ CUPS WHITE SUGAR
- 1½ STICKS MARGARINE
- 6 TABLESPOONS VANILLA EXTRACT
- 1 TABLESPOON NUTMEG
- 1 TABLESPOON CINNAMON

THIS IS KELLY'S FAVORITE RECIPE. IT GOES GREAT WITH THE TURKEY.

1. Peel the yams and cut each one into 4 large pieces (if you desire smaller pieces, that's fine). *2.* In a large pot, place the yams in enough water to slightly cover the top of the pieces. Bring to a boil. *3.* Add the rest of the ingredients and boil until the liquid looks like maple syrup—thick! *4.* Serve warm. Bon appétit!

SERVES 8 TO 10

Angie's Peach Cobbler

INGREDIENTS

4–6 CUPS SLICED CANNED PEACHES, DRAINED

½ CUP BUTTER OR MARGARINE

1 CUP SUGAR

1 TEASPOON VANILLA EXTRACT

1 TEASPOON CINNAMON

1 TEASPOON NUTMEG

1 CUP SELF-RISING FLOUR

1½ CUPS ALL-PURPOSE FLOUR

¾ CUP BUTTER CRISCO SHORTENING

½ CUP COLD WATER

1 DASH SALT

MY NIECE ANGIE HAS MANY TALENTS. NOT ONLY CAN SHE USE GLITTER AND RHINESTONES TO MAKE A GREAT PAIR OF SHOES INTO A ONE-OF-A-KIND ORIGINAL BUT SHE ALSO BAKES A DELICIOUS PEACH COBBLER. WHEN SHE HAS THE TIME, SHE'LL COOK IT FOR US ALL.

1. Preheat the oven to 375 degrees. *2.* To make the filling: In a saucepan, combine the peaches, butter, sugar, vanilla extract, cinnamon, and nutmeg. Bring to a boil over medium heat and mix well. Remove from the heat and set it aside. *3.* To make the crust: Place the flour, salt, and Crisco in a large mixing bowl. Cut the shortening into the flour until the mixture resembles small peas. Add the ice water and work the dough into a ball. *4.* Roll the dough flat with a rolling pin until the dough is thin (about ⅛ of an inch thick). *5.* Pour the peach filling into a rectangular casserole dish. *6.* Tear one fourth of the dough into smaller pieces. Scatter the pieces over the filling and mix them in well. *7.* Cut the remaining dough into ½-inch strips, and place them diagonally and vertically over the filling, leaving the strips ½ inch apart. *8.* Bake for 30 to 40 minutes or until crust is golden brown. It's the perfect finish to any meal. SERVES 6 TO 8.

Enjoy!

DC FOOD QUIZ

1 Give this girl two drumsticks and a wing from Popeyes chicken and she's a happy camper.

_____

2 This girl eats everything in small portions. She'll pick five things she likes off the menu and eat a little bit of everything until she's full.

_____

3 This girl is the experimental one when it comes to food. She's the one who says, "Let's try sushi." "Let's have octopus." She'll try any food once. Sometimes we look at her and say, "Girl, you're on your own. I'm not eating that."

_____

ANSWERS: 1. BEYONCÉ 2. MICHELLE 3. KELLY

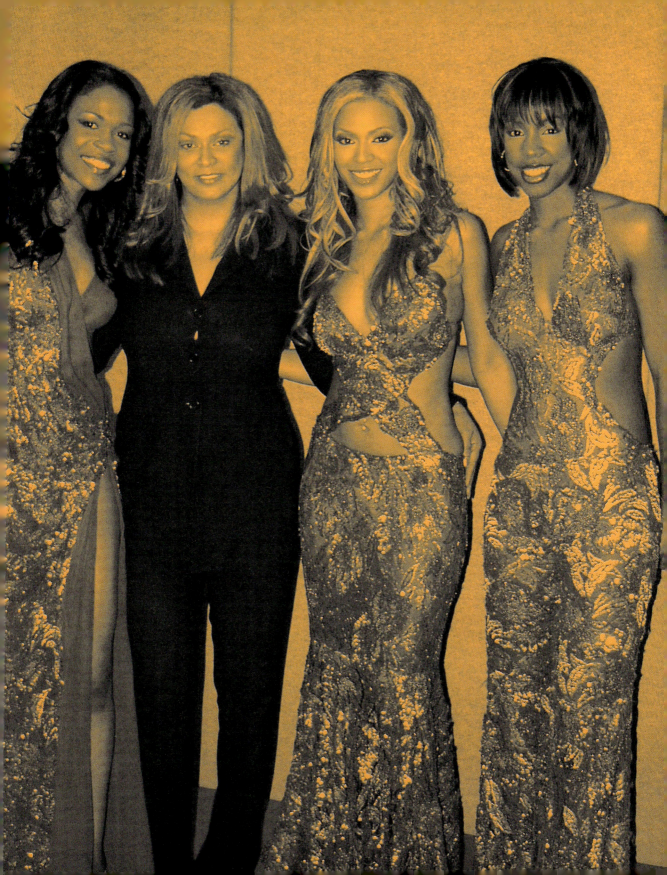

PHOTOGRAPHY CREDITS

Courtesy of Zoë Alexander: 38

© Mark Allan/Globe Photos, Inc.: 6–7, 15, 65 (lower right), 90

© Fitzroy Barrett/Globe Photos, Inc., 2001: xiii, 19, 44, 122–123 © 2000, 124, 157 (lower right)

Alan Floyd/Music World Entertainment: ii, vi–vii, ix, xi (upper right), xiv, xvi (all photos), xix, xx–xxi, 11 (all photos), 17, 20–21, 24–25, 26, 32, 36–37, 46, 49, 52 (upper left, upper right, and lower right), 53 (upper left and bottom right), 54–55, 57, 62–53, 55 (upper left), 68–69, 70, 78, 81, 82–83, 86 (upper right), 87, 89, 92–93, 95, 98, 99, 100–101, 103, 104–105, 108–109, 110, 112, 115, 116, 117, 118–119, 121, 127, 128, 131 (all photos), 132, 134–135, 138, 139, 141, 142, 146 (all photos), 148–149, 151, 152, 154–155, 156 (all photos), 157 (upper left, upper right, and lower left), 158–159, 161, 163, 165 (lower right), 167, 169 (all photos), 172, 174, 176, 177, 182, 183 (bottom), 184–185, 188, 189, 201

© Ed Gellar/Globe Photos, Inc., 2001: 42, 84 © 2000

Courtesy of Tina Knowles: v, xi, xii, 53 (upper right), 133

© Henry McGee/Globe Photos, Inc., 2001: 22, 30–31 © 2000, 74 © 2000, 86 (upper left), 96 © 2000, 145 © 2000

© Alec Michael/Globe Photos, Inc., 2001: 71

Courtesy of Music World Entertainment: 3, 58, 77, 107, 114

© Nina Prommer/Globe Photos, Inc., 2001: 12, 43 © 2000, 52 (lower left) © 2000, 60

© Andrea Renault/Globe Photos, Inc., 2001: 35, 50, 136–137

© Tom Rodriguez/Globe Photos, Inc., 2000: 29

Courtesy of Matthew Rolston: 8

© Lisa Rose/Globe Photos, Inc., 1999: 4

© Milan Ryba/Globe Photos, Inc., 2000: 41

© Jeff Spicer/Globe Photos, Inc.: 72–73

Courtesy of Rod Spicer: 34, 45, 66

Ronald Thomas/Music World Entertainment: 165 (upper right and lower left), 166, 170 (all photos), 179 (all photos), 180, 183 (upper and middle), 187, 190, 193, 195, 197, 205

RESOURCES

Accessories

- AGATHA PARIS
nationwide locations
1.800.777.7595

- JENNIFER KAUFMAN
131 N. La Cienega Boulevard
West Hollywood, CA 90048
1.310.854.1058
www.jenniferkaufman.com

- LORRAINE SCHWARTZ
580 Fifth Avenue
New York, NY 10036

- MIMI SO JEWELERS
580 Fifth Avenue
New York, NY 10036
1.212.354.1407

- SAVVY ACCESSORIES
6701 Harwin Street, #110
Houston, TX 77036
1.713.952.0358

- ShopnOir
248 Mott Street
New York, NY 10012
1.212.966.6868

Clothing

- ARDEN B.
www.ardenb.com
1.800.735.7325

- BCBG
www.bcbg.com
1.888.636.2224

- BEBE
www.bebe.com
1.877.BEBE.777

- BOB MACKIE
545 Madison Ave, 4th Fl.
New York, NY 10022

- CACHÉ
www.cache.com
1.800.788.CACHE (2224)

- DOLCE & GABBANA
816 Madison Avenue
New York, NY 10021
1.212.249.4100
www.dolcegabbana.com

- EXPRESS
www.expressfashion.com
1.614.415.4633

- NEIMAN MARCUS
www.neimanmarcus.com
1.800.825.8000

- SAKS FIFTH AVENUE
www.saks.com
1.800.322.7257

Fabrics

- HIGH FASHION FABRICS
3101 Louisiana Street
Houston, TX 77006
1.713.528.7299

- HOME TEXTILES
Contact: Maria
3802 Fondren Road
Houston, TX 77063
1.713.784.4597

- SOUTHERN IMPORTS
4825 San Jacinto
Houston, TX 77004
1.713.524.8236

- TRADING FAIR
5515 S. Loop East
Houston, TX 77096
1.713.731.1111

Shoes

- GIUSEPPE ZANNOTTI
Available at Saks Fifth
Avenue stores
1.800.322.7257

- JIMMY CHOO
645 Fifth Avenue
New York, NY 10022
1.212.593.0800
www.jimmychoo.com

- MANOLO BLAHNIK
31 W. 54th Street
New York, NY 10019
1.212.582.3007

- PETIT PETON
27 W. 8th St.
New York, NY 10011
1.212.677.3730

- VERSACE
www.versace.com
1.212.465.1200

Home Furnishings

- ACCENT FURNITURE
2950 Fondren Road
Houston, TX 77063
1.713.785.3702

- LIFESTYLE FURNITURE
3190 Fondren Road
Houston, TX 77063
1.713.782.2288

- AFRICAN TREASURES
Lloyd Gite
1.713.880.4975

- NOELLE FURNITURE
2727 South West Freeway
Houston, TX 77063
1.713.784.4597

Tableware

- MARSHALLS
1.800.marshalls

- ROSS
www.rossstores.com

- VERSACE
www.versace.com

ACKNOWLEDGMENTS

I'd like to thank the following people:

God for everything I am.

Mat for, as usual, convincing me that I could do this.

Kelly, Beyoncé, Michelle, and Solange for making my clothes look good.

All my girls: Vernelle, Angie Phea, Cheryl, Stephanie, Yvette, Wanda, Selena, and Flo.

Reggie Wells and Billy B; I love you.

Hymie, who totally understands my vision. You're a genius; I love you.

Angie Beyince; Ty Hunter and Lee Bryant—my right hand. I love you.

Columbia Records; Quincy, Michelle Welch, and St. John's Church.

Zoë Alexander for putting up with my schedule and for being so talented.

Anissa Gordon; Alan Floyd and Ronald Thomas—the bombest photographers.

Thanks to Matthew Rolston.

Regan Books and Renée Iwaszkiewicz: Thanks for your patience and support.

And Wyclef Jean for saying, "Yo ma, you need to style them all the time."

Zoë Alexander thanks:

Mom and Dad for instilling a strong work ethic in me at a young age.

Irami—you're next.

David Dunton, my fantastic lit agent, for helping me hit the first pitch out of the park.

Renée Iwaszkiewicz at ReganBooks for burning as much midnight oil as I did on this.

Judith Regan for being an inspiration.

Nevin Martell for everything. You're a rock star!

Bill Maher for being like a crazy uncle to me and for all the wisdom you've imparted to me over the years.

Special thanks to the following people for their insight into Tina: Mathew, Solange, and Beyoncé Knowles, Kelly Rowland, Michelle Williams, and the entire "Destiny's Child family" including Angela Beyince, Kim Burse, and Ty Hunter for making me feel like "the fifth Beatle." Dieter Esch at Wilhelmina Agency, Yvette Noel-Schure and Matheu Hinton from Columbia Records, Anissa Gordon, Maisha Harrell, Joe Sutton and Renee Louis, Alan Floyd from Music World, Reggie Wells, and Vernelle Jackson.

Last but not least, extra special thanks to Tina Knowles. From the Versace boutique in NYC to the Bentley showroom in Houston (and all exotic locales in between), the lessons I learned from you while participating in the time-honored traditions of shopping and "girl talk" about life, love, family, and style will stay with me forever. God bless.